INTRODUCTION TO HEALTH CAREERS

INTRODUCTION
TO HEALTH
CAREERS

SABRINA HUTTON EDMOND

To order additional copies of this book, contact:
Xlibris Corporation
1-888-795-4274
www.Xlibris.com
Orders@Xlibris.com
98329

Contents

Exploring Health-Care Careers

Course Title: Exploring Health Service Careers
Instructor: Mrs. S. Edmond

Course Description: This course is designed to give the student an overview of the various entry-level occupations and work sites available in the health-care field. It will also provide them with pre-entry skills to help them when they take courses for the entry-level health-care field of their choice.

Course Objectives: When you complete this course, you will

1. have an overview of what the term *health-care team* refers to;
2. have a basic understanding of human anatomy and physiology;
3. have a general knowledge of health-care terminology;
4. be familiar with the skills, education, and duties of at least two health-care careers;
5. be knowledgeable of universal precautions in the health-care field;
6. be aware of the various employment environments in the health-care field (hospital, HMOs, private offices, insurance offices, convalescence homes, etc.);
7. perform basic vital functions;
8. take basic vital functions;
9. be knowledgeable of common communicable diseases;
10. write a résumé and generic letter of application for entry-level employment in the health career field of your choice.

Course Outline and Objectives

Course: Health Science
Phase: 1
Description: Introduction to the Body Systems

I. General Objectives

The student who successfully completes this phase will be able to do the following:

1. Identify the ten body systems.

    a. The skeletal system
    b. The muscular system
    c. The digestive system
    d. The circulatory system
    e. The respiratory system
    f. The nervous system
    g. The integumentary system
    h. The urinary system
    i. The endocrine system
    j. The reproductive system

2. Demonstrate understanding of the major functions of each of the ten body systems.
3. Complete each unit worksheets.
4. Define *body system*.
5. Define the major organs in each body system.

II. Performance Objectives

This phase consists of ten units. For each unit, the student will

1. read the instructor-developed reading materials for each unit,
2. actively participate in lecture/discussions,
3. complete each unit worksheet,
4. complete each unit test with a minimum score of 60%,
5. complete the final phase evaluation test with a minimum score of 70% or better.

III. Instructional Strategies

The instructional strategies will include the use of various commonly acknowledged teaching techniques, including lectures, class discussions, quizzes, demonstrations, individualized instructions, group instructions, and guest speakers when possible. Audio and video materials will be used when available. Students will be encouraged to read outside materials covering the concepts being taught.

IV. Grading System

1. Each unit will have a twenty-question quiz.
2. Each unit quiz will carry the same weight as far as grading is concerned.
3. Quiz grades will be as follows:

90% to 100%	A
80% to 85%	B
70% to 75%	C
60% to 65%	D
Lower than 60%	No Pass

4. A final evaluation quiz will cover all ten units. It will weigh as 50% of the final phase score.

    The final evaluation quiz will be graded as follows:

    90% to 100%   A

    80% to 85%   B

    70% to 75%   C

    60% to 65%   D

    Lower than 60%   No Pass

5. The final grade will be based on the average score of the ten unit tests combined with the final evaluative test scores.

V. Evaluation

1. The final grade will be based on the average score of the ten unit tests combined with the score of the final evaluation test.

2. To pass this phase, the student must meet the following standards:

    a. The student must receive a minimum score of 60% in each of the unit test.

    b. The students must receive an average score of 70% in the ten unit tests.

    c. The student must receive a minimum score of 70% in the final evaluation test.

    d. The student must achieve an average score of 70% in the ten unit tests combined with the final exam.

VI. Retaking Test

1. Students may retake the test during the last week of the quarter if they

   a. score less than 60% in any unit test,
   b. have an average score of less than 70% on the unit test,
   c. score less than 70% on the final evaluation test.

2. Students failing to meet the minimum standard of a 70% average score will retake the class.

1. The skeletal system can be compared to a _____.

    a. car
    b. movie
    c. telephone
    d. horse
    e. none of the above

2. The basic framework of the body is called the _____.

    a. cardiac system
    b. endocrine system
    c. skeletal system
    d. muscular system
    e. none of the above

3. The muscular system can be seen as the body's _____.

    a. framework
    b. movers
    c. workers
    d. digestive system
    e. none of the above

4. Muscles work in _____ by pulling.

    a. sections
    b. place
    c. composition
    d. pairs
    e. none of the above

5. Muscles compose nearly _____ of our body weight.

    a. 95%

    b. 90%

    c. 9%

    d. 25%

    e. none of the above

6. Bones are composed of _____.

    a. tissues

    b. blood vessels

    c. nerves

    d. all of the above

    e. none of the above

7. The body has _____ kinds of muscle tissues.

    a. 2

    b. 4

    c. 6

    d. 8

    e. none of the above

8. Bones are connected by _____.

    a. ligaments

    b. nerves

    c. muscles

    d. joints

    e. none of the above

9. Smooth muscles are _____ muscles.

    a. involuntary
    b. voluntary
    c. the strongest
    d. all of the above
    e. none of the above

10. Immovable joints are _____.

    a. fibrous
    b. cartilaginous
    c. synovial
    d. skeletal
    e. none of the above

11. Skeletal muscles are _____ muscles (controlled by will).

    a. involuntary
    b. reflex
    c. smooth muscles
    d. not controlled by consciousness
    e. none of the above

12. Freely movable joints are _____.

    a. fibrous
    b. cartilaginous
    c. synovial
    d. skeletal
    e. none of the above

13. Cardiac muscles pump blood to the body's _____ system.

    a. skeletal
    b. heart
    c. muscle
    d. circulatory
    e. none of the above

14. The main function of the cranial skeleton is to protect the _____.

    a. eyes
    b. brain
    c. both *a* and *b*
    d. hair follicles
    e. heart

15. All muscles _____.

    a. bend
    b. pull
    c. pump blood
    d. move bones
    e. none of the above

16. The weight of the cranial skeleton, trunk, and upper limbs is supported by the _____.

    a. spinal cord
    b. skull
    c. pelvic bone
    d. lower limbs
    e. none of the above

17. Every bone or organ in the body that moves, pumps, or pushes is controlled by a/an _____.

    a. skeletal muscle
    b. voluntary muscle
    c. smooth muscle
    d. pair of muscles
    e. none of the above

18. Involuntary muscles are not controlled by _____.

    a. blood
    b. organs
    c. will
    d. tissue
    e. none of the above

19. Functions of the bones include _____.

    a. the production of blood cells
    b. the facilitation of skeletal movement
    c. the storing of calcium
    d. all of the above
    e. none of the above

20. When muscles pull, this is called _____.

    a. contraction
    b. pullation
    c. circulation
    d. will power
    e. ventilation

Classroom Contract

My signature below acknowledges that I, the student, agree to do the following:

1. Come to all classes.
2. Be on time.
3. Participate in all class activities.
4. Complete all assignments.
5. Pass all tests with a minimum score of 70%.
6. Come to class prepared.
7. Conduct myself as an adult.

     _____   _____

             Student signature   Date

My signature below acknowledges that I, the teacher, will do the following:

1. Treat each student fairly.
2. Provide the student with accurate information.
3. Assure that the classroom is conducive for learning.
4. Answer all questions to the best of my ability.
5. Make the class curriculum interesting and encourage your participation.

     _____   _____

                 Instructor   Date

Interview Log

Date _____

Name _____
Age _____
Job or trade _____
Number of children _____

Why are you taking this class?

What do you expect to learn?

Do you know of any jobs or careers that are available in the health science field?

Introduction to Health-Care Careers

Since the earliest days of mankind, the health-care provider has been one of the most respected individuals in a community. The health-care provider has always been a dedicated and caring person whose number one objective has been to provide their patients the best medical care available. Medicine has come a long way since ancient times; however, its practitioners still have one goal in common—the preservation of life. From the witch doctor to Hippocrates to today's doctors, the health and well-being of each patient are what all health-care workers strive to maintain as part of a health-care team.

As modern medicine improves and expands, so do health-care careers. The first doctors worked by themselves, often using family members of the sick patient to perform some of the menial duties such as boiling water, cleaning an area, making bandages, etc. However, as medicine became more complicated, the doctors found the need to have nurses who were trained in patient care, disinfection, and asepsis. The more technical medicine becomes, the more health careers come into being. Improvement in laboratory techniques brought on the advent of the phlebotomist. Large hospitals, medical insurance companies, and HMOs brought about the need for billing and insurance clerks.

The quest for new and better medicine made it impossible for pharmacists to fill all their prescriptions, therefore requiring them to hire assistants, more commonly referred to as pharmacy technicians. The discovery of ether as an anesthetic made way for the anesthesiologist. In fact, the more we learn about medicine and health care, the more employment opportunities open in health care.

Today, employment in the health-care service field is one of the fastest-growing segments in America's job market. The need for nonprofessional personnel is at its greatest levels in history. There is a great demand for nurses, medical receptionists, front and back office workers, billing clerks, x-ray technicians, dental assistants, pharmacy technicians, phlebotomists, laboratory assistants, sanitary engineers, and various other health-care professionals.

Because of the expanding health-care needs of a growing population with increasing numbers of elderly people, employment in medical care services will greatly increase in the years to come. The Bureau of Labor Statistics has revised its labor force projections for the 1990s. Listed among the fastest-growing occupations are a number of health-related careers. Actually, the health industry is one of the largest in the United States.

Some jobs today didn't exist a few years ago. For example, many jobs have resulted from the discovery of the x-ray. Today, there are even more advanced uses for x-rays. Computerized tomographic scanners are providing new jobs.

These scanners are x-ray machines that can take pictures of a section of the inside of the body without shadows from other sections interfering. Since computers are being used to study and interpret information from laboratories, people who know about them are also needed in the health field.

How should you prepare for a health career? There is no single answer to this question because there are so many different careers. Since there is a wide choice of careers, the length of time needed and the place of preparation vary. For instance, other jobs have a training period that begins after high school and lasts for several weeks or months. Still others require several years of professional training. Being a physician requires a college degree in addition to years of specialized training.

The health careers that require the least amount of formal education are called entry-level careers. Some entry-level health careers are those of surgical technicians, EEG technologists, EKG technologists, respiratory therapy technicians, clinical laboratory assistants, dietetic technicians, and medical assistants.

Intermediate-level careers in health require an associate degree, which can be earned in two years. Some of the intermediate-level health careers are those of cytotechnologists, dental hygienists, pediatric assistants, radiation therapy technologists, licensed practical nurses, and physical therapy assistants.

Professional-level careers in health usually require a four-year college degree although several of these professions require additional years of education, training, and experience. Some higher-level health careers include those of medical technologists, speech pathologists, health educators, veterinarians, occupational therapists, registered nurses, physical therapists, and physicians.

This course is designed to provide you with information to help guide you toward one of the many health-care service jobs in demand and to gear you toward being an effective, efficient, and knowledgeable member of a health-care team.

Minimal Skill Requirements for Health-Care Careers

Whether the students will be working in a medical office, HMO, outpatient clinic, convalescence home, or hospital, most entry-level health careers require the following minimal skills:

- Minimal typing skills
- Computer literacy
- Tenth-grade or higher reading level
- Interpersonal-relation skills
- Communication skills
- Writing proficiency
- Basic math skills
- Basic accounting skills
- Basic knowledge of anatomy and physiology
- High school diploma or GED certificate
- Knowledge of basic vital signs
- Knowledge of metric system
- Knowledge of basic medical terminology
- Knowledge of universal precautions
- Knowledge of medical ethics
- Knowledge of medical law
- Basic filing skills
- Knowledge of first aid and CPR
- Telephone communication techniques
- Preparation of charts
- Preparation of correspondence

Some Other Careers in the Health Field

Biomedical equipment technician
Computer programmer
Dental laboratory technician
Dentist
Dietitian (nutritionist)
Dietetic technician
Emergency medical technician
Health educator
Histologic technician
Inhalation therapy technician
Medical librarian
Medical social worker
Registered nurse (RN)
Nursing aide
Optometric technician

Osteopath
Podiatrist (chiropodist)
Prosthetist and orthotist
Clinical psychologist
Medical laboratory technician
Industrial hygienist
Food technologist
Public health engineer
Noise technician
Nurse practitioner
Medical record technician
Optician
Optometrist
Pharmacist

Sabrina Hutton Edmond

Student's Interview Sheet

Date of interview _____

Interviewer _____

Interviewee _____

Age of interviewee: [] 14-18 [] 19-21 [] 21-over

Highest grade completed in school _____

Why are you taking this class? _____

_____

_____

_____

What are your hobbies? _____

_____

_____

_____

Have you ever worked in the health-care field? [] Yes [] No

If yes, where? _____

_____

What health-care career/s are you interested in pursuing?

1. _____

2. _____

3. _____

Why would you make a good health-care worker?

_____

_____

_____

Health Careers

Orientation Quiz

1. After completing this course, you will receive _____.

    a. a CNA license
    b. a medical receptionist certificate
    c. a medical pin
    d. all of the above
    e. none of the above

2. After completing this course, you will _____.

    a. be a certified nurse assistant
    b. be a medical secretary
    c. be a dental assistant
    d. all of the above
    e. none of the above

3. After completing this course, you will _____.

    a. know the requirements needed to be a phlebotomist
    b. know the requirements needed to be a dental assistant
    c. know the requirements needed to be an x-ray technician
    d. all of the above
    e. none of the above

4. After completing this course, you will _____.

    a. receive a phlebotomy certificate
    b. receive a medical nursing pin
    c. receive a typing certificate
    d. all of the above
    e. none of the above

5. After completing this course, you will _____.

    a. receive a health-care certificate
    b. receive a CPR certificate
    c. all of the above
    d. none of the above

6. This course is best designed for _____.

    a. students interested in becoming doctors or RNs
    b. students interested in medicine
    c. students wanting to become medical office workers
    d. students interested in health careers
    e. students interested in pharmacology

7. A medical assistant would be considered _____.

    a. entry level
    b. intermediate
    c. professional
    d. none of the above
    e. all of the above

8. Which health career requires the least amount of education?

    a. physical therapy
    b. EKG technologist
    c. cytotechnologist
    d. none of the above
    e. all of the above

9. Medicine over the last hundred years _____.

    a. has made few changes
    b. has remained the same
    c. has reached its limits
    d. has changed dramatically
    e. has shown little progress since Hippocrates

10. A phlebotomist _____.

    a. must study for five years
    b. is an entry-level health-care technician
    c. is an intermediate-level health-care technician
    d. must take the Hippocratic oath
    e. is a professional-level health-care technician

The Reproductive System

Unit Test 10

1. How many chromosomes are there in a human body cell?

    a. 122
    b. 12
    c. 23
    d. 46
    e. none of the above

2. How many chromosomes are there in a human sex cell?

    a. 122
    b. 12
    c. 23
    d. 46
    e. none of the above

3. Female sex cells are called _____.

    a. spermatozoa
    b. gonads
    c. ova
    d. meiosis
    e. none of the above

4. Male sex cells are called _____.

    a. spermatozoa
    b. gonads
    c. ova
    d. meiosis
    e. none of the above

5. Gonads are _____.

   a. female sex organs
   b. male
   c. both male and female sex organs
   d. asexual organs
   e. none of the above

6. Which of the following is a sex cell?

   a. spermatozoa
   b. ova
   c. germ cells
   d. all of the above
   e. none of the above

7. Sex glands that produce germ cells and hormones are called _____.

   a. gonads
   b. Cowper's
   c. prostate glands
   d. all of the above
   e. none of the above

8. The male sex gland that produces germ cells is the _____.

   a. Cowper's gland
   b. testes
   c. testosterone
   d. ovaries
   e. none of the above

9. The female sex gland that produces germ cells is the _____.

    a. Cowper's glands

    b. testes

    c. testosterone

    d. ovaries

    e. none of the above

10. The Cowper's gland secretes _____ into semen.

    a. germ cells

    b. mucus

    c. spermatozoa

    d. alkaline

    e. none of the above

11. The prostate glands secrete _____ into semen.

    a. germ cells

    b. mucus

    c. spermatozoa

    d. alkaline

    e. none of the above

12. The penis is filled with blood to allow _____.

    a. intercourse

    b. urination

    c. hormone production

    d. development of spermatozoa

    e. none of the above

13. Female gonads are called _____.

    a. ovaries

    b. testes

    c. vagina

    d. uterus

    e. none of the above

14. All except for _____ is a sex hormone.

    a. testosterone

    b. estrogen

    c. progesterone

    d. estradiol

    e. ovum

15. _____ is a male sex hormone.

    a. testosterone

    b. ovum

    c. progesterone

    d. seminal fluid

    e. none of the above

16. The female sex cell is called a/an _____.

    a. ova

    b. cilia

    c. vaginal fluid

    d. all of the above

    e. none of the above

17. The female oviducts are also referred to as _____.

    a. ovum

    b. fallopian tubes

    c. ova

    d. all of the above

    e. none of the above

18. The oviducts move the ovum to the uterus in _____ days.

    a. 1

    b. 7

    c. 3

    d. 4

    e. none of the above

19. A fetus grows to maturity in the _____.

    a. ovaries

    b. urethra

    c. uterus

    d. vagina

    e. none of the above

20. The female reproductive system is cyclical. How often does it take place?

    a. for 10 days each month

    b. once each month

    c. once each year

    d. once each week

    e. none of the above

Introduction to Health Science

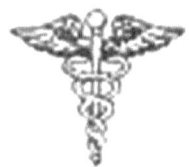

Unit 1

Communicable Diseases

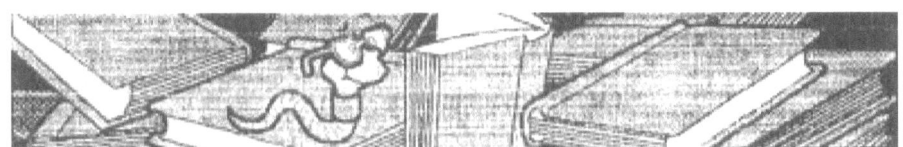

Communicable Diseases

A *disease* is a medical condition characterized by specific abnormal changes in the body's functions. A disease presents a group of *clinical* signs and symptoms and laboratory findings *peculiar* to the body. A disease is usually tangible, has an organic cause, and is often *measurable*. Illness is often confused with disease; however, illness is generally *individualized* and personal and most commonly associated with pain, suffering, and distress. Its cause has no organic explanation. A disease is often accompanied by illness, thus further causing confusion of the medical condition.

There are various kinds of diseases. In this lesson, we will be discussing some commonly occurring communicable diseases. These diseases spread from person to person. All communicable diseases are caused by *pathogens*. Pathogens are microscopic living things that cause disease. *Bacteria*, a one-celled microscopic pathogen, is responsible for many diseases. A *virus* is another pathogen that causes communicable diseases. A virus, like bacteria, is microscopic; however, it *multiplies* and grows inside the body's cells. Unlike bacteria, a virus is not a cell, nor does it contain cells.

Bacteria and viruses are almost everywhere. They do not cause diseases until they enter the human tissue. Once they enter the human tissue, pathogens spread by means of *transmission*. Transmission can be made directly or indirectly. Direct transmission takes place *via* body contact, secretion, or discharge. Indirect transmission takes place via airborne methods, insect contact, food and drink contamination, and contaminated objects.

Many communicable diseases are life threatening. In some cases, immunization is available to prevent diseases; this will be discussed in more detail in unit G.

The communicable diseases that we will be divided into five transmission groups. Although some of these diseases can be transmitted in more than one way, they have been grouped according to their most common means of transmission.

Although each communicable disease has its own distinct set of symptoms, there are some symptoms that are common among most of them. These symptoms include sore throat, fever, swollen glands, runny nose, red eyes, yellow eyes and skin, coughs, chest pains, breathing difficulties, muscle pains, headache, nausea, vomiting, and fatigue. The common symptoms among most sexually transmitted diseases have their own symptoms. These symptoms include discharge from the sex organ, painful blisters, burning, redness of the sex organ, painful sores in or around the sex organ, rash, fever, and in some cases, no symptoms at all. Knowledge of communicable diseases is especially essential to pregnant women because these diseases can affect or even infect the unborn child.

As stated earlier, communicable diseases are all caused by bacteria or viruses and are transmitted directly or indirectly. On the following pages, I have divided them into five groups based on their most common mode of transmission.

Communicable Diseases Grouped According to Transmission

1. Transmitted by sexual contact

    a. Syphilis
    b. Gonorrhea
    c. Chlamydia
    d. Herpes
    e. AIDS

2. Transmitted by air

    a. Tuberculosis
    b. Leprosy

3. Transmitted by bacteria

    a. Whooping cough
    b. Pneumonia
    c. Strep throat
    d. Mumps
    e. Meningitis
    f. Measles
    g. Influenza
    h. Diphtheria

4. Transmitted by contact with blood

    a. Tetanus
    b. Hepatitis B
    c. Hepatitis C

5. Transmitted by contact with feces and/or urine

    a. Hepatitis A
    b. Cholera

Communicable diseases transmitted by sexual contact are usually preventable by use of condoms. Syphilis, gonorrhea, and chlamydia are curable. Usually, specific antibiotics are used to cure the above diseases. Herpes at the present time is incurable, yet it is not life threatening, although often painful. AIDS is the deadliest of all these diseases and one of the fastest-growing killers of man today. Like herpes, AIDS is not curable. AIDS may be dormant for as many as eight or more years, but it is almost always terminal.

Communicable diseases transmitted by air are highly contagious. Thanks to modern medicine, the two major airborne communicable diseases are now treatable if diagnosed early. Leprosy, as stated earlier, is curable; however, its treatment is long and complicated. Tuberculosis, though once always fatal, is now curable, and its treatment period lasts approximately six months. New strains of tuberculosis have been observed recently and do not respond well to standard treatments; however, new drugs have been effective in their cure.

Blood-transmitted diseases that you could be exposed to are tetanus, hepatitis B, and hepatitis C. Several of the sexually transmitted diseases can also be transmitted by blood contact. *Hepatitis* means inflammation of the liver. Hepatitis B virus, commonly known as HBV, is the major infectious blood-borne hazard you could face. If you become infected with HBV, you may suffer from flu-like symptoms becoming so severe that you may require hospitalization. You may be totally unaware of any symptom at all, yet you are infected.

Your blood, saliva, and other body fluids can be infectious. You can spread a virus to your mate, your family members, and even your unborn child. HBV is known to severely damage your liver and lead to cirrhosis and certain death.

Other communicable diseases are caused by bacteria. The diseases are usually transmitted by *secretion* or *discharge* from the nose, throat, mouth, or glands. Diseases caused by bacteria include pneumonia, influenza, measles, diphtheria, strep throat, mumps, whooping cough, and meningitis. Some can be prevented by immunization; measles, mumps, whooping cough and diphtheria are examples. In most cases, *antibiotics* will effectively combat these contagious bacterial diseases. Antibiotics are chemical substances produced by living cells to kill or arrest the growth of pathogens.

Feces is human or animal waste that is usually excreted from the bowels. Urine is fluid and other dissolved substances excreted from the body through the urethra. Two of the most dangerous diseases known to man, hepatitis A and cholera, are caused by human contact with feces or urine. With these two diseases, the best course is prevention. Thus, it is important to observe general sterilization and sanitation practices.

Communicable diseases are also categorized as being epidemic, endemic, or pandemic. *Epidemic* refers to many people in a certain region acquiring a disease. *Endemic* refers to a disease being found continuously in a specific region. *Pandemic* refers to a disease that is prevalent throughout the country, continent, or world.

Universal Precautions for Communicable Diseases

To help prevent the spread of communicable diseases, universal precautions have been introduced. Some blood-borne diseases like AIDS and hepatitis are incurable and cause the greatest concern; however, under universal precautions, all communicable diseases are treated as if they are incurable.

The universal precautions include the following:

1. Assume that all body fluids have the potential for transmission of disease.
2. Wear gloves, gowns, and protective goggles when helping someone who has a communicable disease.
3. Wash hands thoroughly and frequently.
4. Never recap needles.
5. Protect your mucous membranes and broken skin.
6. Treat all waste and laundry as if contaminated.

To learn more about a particular disease that we have discussed, I would encourage you to utilize the library or a good encyclopedia. Notice that most communicable diseases are preventable. Cleanliness and precaution, especially when around others, are the best methods of prevention. Also, taking care of your health is important. A person with a strong immune system is less likely to contract a communicable disease than someone who has let their immune system weaken.

Common Bacterial and Viral Communicable Diseases

* Bacterial
- Viral

Disease	Cause
Syphilis	*
Gonorrhea	*
Chlamydia	*
Herpes	-
AIDS	-
Tuberculosis	*
Leprosy	*
Whooping cough	*
Pneumonia	*/-
Strep throat	*
Mumps	-
Meningitis	*
Measles	-
Influenza	-
Diphtheria	*
Tetanus	*
Hepatitis A	-
Hepatitis B	-
Hepatitis C	-
Cholera	*
Legionnaire's disease	*
Chicken pox	-
Ringworm	*
Common cold	-
Encephalitis	-

Unit 1 Worksheet

Communicable
Disease

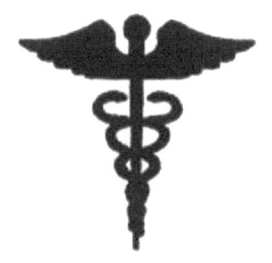

1. A _____ is a medical condition characterized by abnormal changes in the body's function.
2. An _____, unlike a disease, has no organic cause and is usually associated with pain, suffering, and/or distress.
3. All _____ diseases are caused by pathogens.
4. Bacteria and virus are both _____.
5. A one-celled pathogen that causes communicable diseases is called a

    _____.
6. A _____ is a pathogen that is not a cell, nor does it contain cells.
7. Pathogens spread by means of _____.
8. The transmission of pathogens can be made _____ or _____.
9. Transmission of a disease by body contact is an example of _____ transmission.
10. Transmission of a disease by airborne sources is an example of _____ transmission.
11. Syphilis is commonly transmitted via _____.
12. Tuberculosis is an example of an _____ transmitted disease.
13. Influenza is commonly transmitted by a _____.
14. Hepatitis B is commonly transmitted by contact with _____.
15. Cholera is commonly transmitted by contact with _____ or urine.
16. _____ can be used to prevent infection by sexually transmitted diseases.
17. HBV is an acronym for _____.
18. The body organ most often affected by HBV is the _____.
19. _____ is human or animal waste excreted from the bowels.
21. _____ is fluid or dissolved substances excreted by the way of the urethra.
22. A strong _____ system is helpful in the prevention of contracting communicable diseases.

23. Antibiotics will not combat communicable diseases caused by
_____.

24. A disease that is prevalent throughout the world is said to be
_____.

25. List the six universal precautions for a person's protection against
communicable diseases.

a. _____

b. _____

c. _____

d. _____

e. _____

f. _____

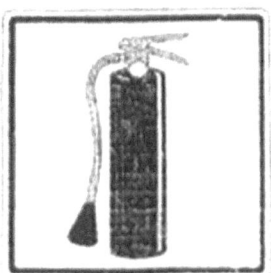

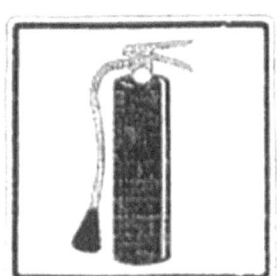

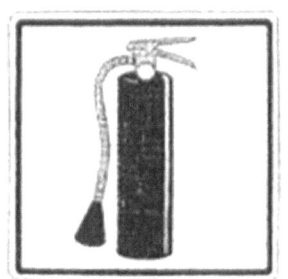

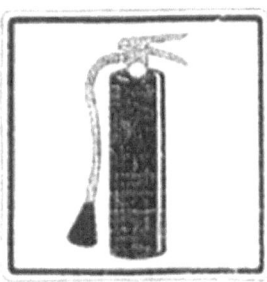

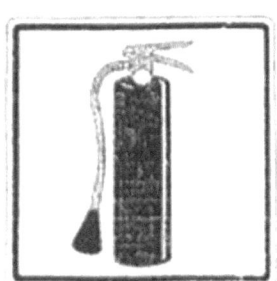

Safety for Health-Care Careers

Key Terms

MSDS
oxygen
triage
incident
5 Ws
disaster
evacuation
prevention
universal precaution
pathogens
microorganism
RACE
infection

Objectives: The student will identify hazardous situations as they relate to fire, electricity, chemicals, and oxygen; be knowledgeable of a triage disaster plan; identify evacuation plans; know the universal precautions; identify the four types of fire extinguishers; know the meaning of RACE; and read an MSDS.

Table of Contents

General Rules for Institutional Safety

When working in a health-care environment, health-care personnel must be careful to guard themselves and their patients against accidents. In the event of an emergency, all health-care personnel may be needed to help evacuate the facility or to transport patients and injured personnel to a secured area. For these reasons, general rules of institutional safety must be observed by all health-care personnel.

Most safety rules are common sense; however, it is sometimes important to review some of them. The list of general rules below is not all-inclusive; however, they will be helpful in making your work environment safe for you, your patients, and your coworkers.

1. Be safety conscious at all times.
2. Avoid running, especially in hallways or on stairs.
3. Use handrails.
4. Be knowledgeable of the international hospital code system, the triage disaster plan codes, and the universal precaution guidelines.
5. Adhere to all safety and warning signs.
6. Be careful that feet and limbs are properly positioned on footrests and armrests.
7. Lock brakes on movable equipment when moving patients on or off such equipment.
8. Remove articles that do not belong on the floor.
9. Wipe up spilled liquids immediately.
10. Wear proper protective equipment and clothing that are appropriate for the work environment.
11. Report lighting and electrical failures, equipment malfunctions, and hazards such as loose or broken tiles, glass, and carpeting.

12. Be knowledgeable of the types of fire retardants.

13. Avoid and report any electrical hazards.

14. Read the MSDS (material safety data sheet) for all chemicals before using them.

15. Make sure that the work area is well ventilated when using chemicals such as paint, poison spray, and fumigants.

Oxygen Safety

When your work environment necessitates the use of oxygen tanks and regulators, be knowledgeable of the precautions used around oxygen. Extra oxygen helps combustion, causing fires to burn more rapidly than they would in normal air.

1. No Smoking: Oxygen in Use signs should be posted in areas where oxygen is being used.
2. Report when the tubing connected to the source of oxygen is not free of kinks.
3. Never smoke in an area where oxygen is being used.
4. Never start a fire in an area where oxygen is being used.
5. Report cigarettes and matches belonging to a patient to the office supervisor.
6. Report any oxygen use that is administered without a physician's order.
7. Report any leaks or suspected leaks in oxygen equipment.
8. Never use oxygen in areas where there are sparks.

Fire Safety

Fire safety involves two primary areas: prevention and action. There are seven major causes of fire:

1. Smoking
2. Matches
3. Electrical malfunctions
4. Chemical reactions
5. Defective heating systems
6. Spontaneous ignition
7. Improper disposal of garbage

For a fire to start, there are three essential elements:

1. Fuel (paper, clothing, building material, etc.)
2. Ignition (heat source [e.g., flame, sparks])
3. Oxygen (the air we breathe)

To prevent fires, the combination of the three elements for starting fires should be avoided at all times. Smoking is the number one cause of fire in health-care facilities. If smoking is allowed in your facility, take the following precautions:

1. Provide ashtrays.
2. Keep ashtrays emptied and free of paper and other combustible materials.
3. Make sure that all emptied materials are fully extinguished.
4. Smoke and allow smoking only in permitted areas.
5. If you are a patient-care personnel, do not allow sedated patients to smoke.
6. Report any violators and violations of the smoking policy to your supervisor.

In the event of a fire, use the RACE system. RACE is an acronym for Remove, Activate, Contain, and Extinguish. To use the RACE system, you must be knowledgeable of your facility's escape routes, evacuation procedures, emergency alarm and telephone locations, and firefighting equipment location and usage.

Using the RACE System

Remove all patients and personnel in the vicinity of the fire.

Activate, alarm, notify other coworkers, and call fire department.

Contain the fire by closing all doors in the immediate area.

Extinguish the fire or allow fire personnel to extinguish the fire.

Choosing a Fire Extinguisher

There are basically four kinds of fire extinguishers, each having a specific use. You should be knowledgeable of the four extinguishers' use. Each type should be clearly labeled, and you should know their locations.

A-rated extinguishers are for paper, wood, and trash fires.

B-rated extinguishers are for liquid (oil, grease) fires.

C-rated extinguishers are for electrical fires.

ABC-rated extinguishers can be used to stop all three kinds of fires.

Fire Safety

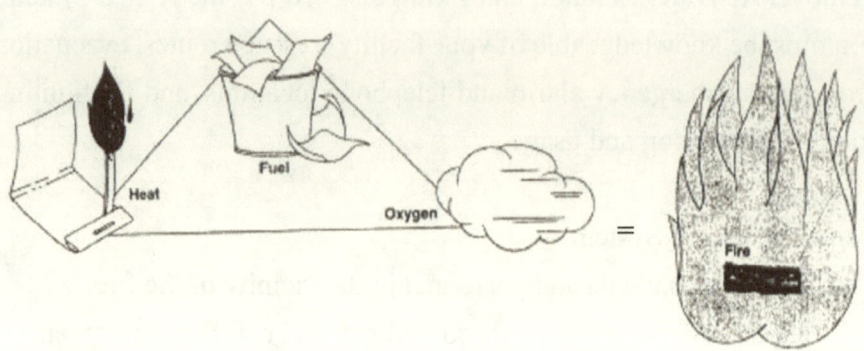

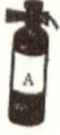 ————————Paper, wood, trash

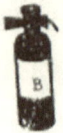 ————————Oil, grease

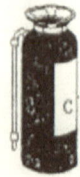 ————————Electrical

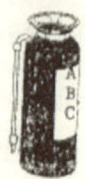 ————————All (paper, wood, trash, oil, grease, electrical)

Electrical Safety

Another major cause of fires, injuries, and deaths at a work site is malfunctioning, misused, improperly connected, or damaged electrical cords and appliances. To prevent electrical-related injuries and shocks, observe the following precautions:

1. Inspect all electrical cords for cuts, bare wires, and frays before plugging them in.
2. Inspect all electrical outlets before inserting a cord.
3. Observe all electrical danger signs.
4. Use a three-pronged grounding plug on all equipment to prevent electrical shock.
5. Do not use a cord when the ground lead (rounded third prong) is broken or removed.
6. Have malfunctioning equipment repaired or replaced.
7. Avoid using lightweight or improper extension cords.
8. Avoid overloading an electrical outlet.
9. Do not use electrical equipment if you receive a shock when touching it.
10. Do not touch an electrical device and a patient at the same time.
11. Be sure that your hands are dry before using electrical equipment.
12. Disconnect electrical cords before you inspect equipment.
13. Do not allow water to come in contact with electrical equipment.
14. Report all electrical hazards to the appropriate personnel.

Chemical Safety

In most health-care facilities, you will have contact with chemicals. Chemicals can cause fires; burns to the skin; irritation of the eyes, skin, hair, and nose; nausea; fainting; and even death when they are used or stored improperly.

When working with or around chemicals, read the MSDS (material safety data sheet). It contains important information about the chemical and its chemical properties. The MSDS provides information regarding your personal safety, advises you of the correct emergency response for spills and contact, gives you information about other environmental concerns for the specific chemical, and tells you how the product should be properly used, stored, and discarded.

Falls

Another preventable accident at the workplace involves falls. Most falls can be prevented by keeping floors clear of debris, wiping spilled liquids immediately, keeping work area well lit, using handrails, and posting safety signs where applicable.

Incident Report Writing

An *incident* can be defined as an unusual event or condition that causes or is likely to cause an accident. As a member of a health-care team, you may observe an incident and will be required to make a written observation of what occurred.

Most health-care facilities have standard forms called incident report forms (see form on page <please insert the correct page no.). It is your responsibility to complete an incident report whenever an incident occurs. All reports should contain the 5 Ws:

1. When did the incident take place (date, time)?
2. What took place?
3. Who were the participants (including the reporters)?
4. Where did the incident take place?
5. Why did the incident occur (if you know)?

Incident reports must be accurate, must contain all the facts, and must be done in a professional manner. They may be included as evidence in a liability suit, worker's compensation compliant, or damage claim. Incident reports should be reviewed by your immediate supervisor before they are filed with the appropriate administrator.

Example of incidents include the following:

1. Patient, employee, or visitor accidents
2. Theft of the facility's property
3. Theft of patient's property
4. Acts of vandalism
5. Fires at the facility
6. Accidents occurring in the facility
7. Spills that cause accidents
8. Assault or battery at the facility

Generic Incident Report

Health-Care Facility Incident Report

1. Report by
    Patient []   Visitor []   Employee []   Other []
2. Date of report _____
3. Name _____Department _____
    Position _____
4. Location where incident occurred _____
5. Time of incident _____ AM _____ PM
6. Describe incident and how accident occurred _____

    _____

    _____

    _____

7. Name/s of witness/es _____

    _____

8. Action taken to prevent reoccurrence _____

    _____

9. Report writer's signature _____ Date _____

    _____

Department director must complete necessary information in duplicate.
Duplicate must be forwarded immediately to the chairman of the safety
committee.

Reviewed by safety committee on _____/_____/_____

Signed _____
         Chairman

A Ten-Step Triage Disaster Plan

If a disaster occurs at a health-care facility, every employee should be aware of the facility's disaster plan and of his or her responsibilities. Each facility should have a written disaster plan that tells the priority for action in the event of a disaster. Each facility's plans are different in terms of who is in charge and which employee is responsible for certain actions to be taken; however, there are some standard procedures that should be adhered to in all triage disaster emergency plans. The ten-step triage plan described in this section should give you an idea of the concept of triage disaster planning. Remember that each facility's plan is different due to logistics. It is important for you to read and know the plan at your facility.

1. Remove the injured from immediate danger. Close doors after removing the injured.
2. Determine level of consciousness of each injured party.
3. Establish airways if needed.
4. Establish signs of breathing and pulse.
5. Treat severe bleeding.
6. Treat poisoning.
7. Treat burns.
8. Treat for shock.
9. Treat fractures.
10. Treat other injuries as needed.

Evacuation Plans

In the event of a fire, threat to the building (bomb), or disaster, you may be required to help evacuate a health-care facility. It is important that every employee knows the escape routes in the facility. These escape routes should be posted throughout the building. Each health-care facility will have its own policies and procedures explaining what to do if you must evacuate the facility. Be knowledgeable of the facility's triage disaster plan; it will be helpful if evacuation is required. *Do* not use the elevators if there is a fire or electrical shorting. It is important that you remain calm during an evacuation; many patients' and visitors' lives may depend on your actions during an evacuation.

A sample evacuation procedure would be the following:

1. Remove patient from immediate danger.
2. Pull nearest emergency alarm.
3. Notify switchboard operator or similar personnel as to the location and the nature of the disaster.
4. Follow the triage disaster plan of your facility and evacuate.

Universal Precautions

When working in a health-care facility or around those who are in need of medical attention, there may be situations in which you have contact with a patient's blood, body fluids, or body substances. These substances may contain pathogens. Pathogens are microorganisms that are harmful and are capable of causing infections.

An infection is a state disease caused by the invasion of pathogens into the body. Pathogens invade the body through the respiratory, urinary, reproductive, and integumentary systems. They can be transported from person to person by breathing, eating, drinking, or contact with animals and insects.

The human body has natural defenses against infections caused by pathogens. We also have developed procedures to help us avoid contracting infections. Since infections can be passed from one person to another, a health-care worker should treat every patient as if he or she were infected.

In 1987, the Center for Disease Control (CDC) issued precautions to prevent the spread of AIDS and other infections. These precautions are referred to as universal precautions—barriers to prevent contact with the patient's blood, body fluids, or body substances. Universal precautions should be used by all health-care personnel. The seven categories of precautions are listed below, and on the following page, you will find a list of the universal precautions. Study them carefully. Your health and that of those around you can be affected by your knowledge of the precautions.

Seven Areas of Precaution

1. Strict   Prevents pathogen spread by direct contact or through the air.

2. Contact   Prevents infection spread by close or direct contact.

3. Respiratory   Prevents spread of pathogens through the air.

4. AFB   Prevents spread of tuberculosis.

5. Enteric   Prevents pathogens being spread through feces.

6. Drainage/Secretion Prevents spread of pathogens from wounds.

7. Blood / Body fluids   Prevents spread of pathogens through direct or indirect contact with blood, body fluids, or body substances.

Universal Precautions

Nursing assistants should adhere to the following precautions when delivering care to all patients. This will decrease the risk of transmission of disease when the infection status of the patient is unknown.

- Gloves must be worn when contact with blood or body fluids (urine, feces, emesis, etc.) is likely, for example, when taking rectal temperatures.
- Gowns or aprons must be worn during procedures or situations when there will be exposure to body fluids, blood, draining wounds, or mucous membranes.
- Mask and protective eyewear or face shield must be worn during procedures that are likely to generate droplets of body specimen, fluids, or blood.
- Gloves are to be worn when collecting all specimens to prevent contamination from body specimen, fluids, or blood.
- Hands must be washed before gloving and after gloves are removed (see hand washing procedures in the chapter on infection control). Hands and other skin surfaces must be washed immediately and thoroughly if contaminated with body fluids or blood and after all patient-care activities.
- Nursing assistants who have open cuts, sores, or dermatitis on their hands must wear gloves for all patient contact.

Material Safety Data Sheet

FORMALEX

PRODUCED BY: S & S COMPANY OF GA., INC.   SOLD BY:

827 Pine Ave./P.O. Box 45

Albany, GA 31702-0045

(912) 435-8394

This MSDS sheet is provided to you pursuant to 29 CFR, 1910.1200, the "OSHA Hazard Communication Standard".

This Data Sheet contains confidential product information as well as information regarding personal safety, emergency response for spills of this product, and other environmental information.

This information is for use in your facility for the intended purpose only, and is not for release to individuals outside of your facility, or to other suppliers for product comparison without our express written consent.

Date Printed: Jul 27, 1993
MSDS Date: 16 JUL 93

= =

SECTION I: PRODUCT IDENTIFICATION
& EMERGENCY INFORMATION

= =

Product Name: FORMALEX   CAS #: MIXTURE

Chemical Name: N/A

Chemical Family: Neutralizer

Formula: PROPRIETARY

???. T. Shipping Name: Cleaning Comp Liquid

Hazard Classification: N/A   U.N. Number: N/A

= =

Emergency Telephone Numbers: S & S Company of Georgia, Inc.
(912) 435-8394

= =

SECTION II: PHYSICAL/ENVIRONMENTAL DATA

= =

PHYSICAL DATA:

Bailing Point @ 760mm Hg : 144   Freezing Point: N/D

Specific Gravity (H20=1) : 1.116   Water Solubility: 100%

Vapor Pressure @ 20 C.   : N/D   Vapor Density, (Air=1): N/D

Volatiles—% by Volume   : 0%   Evaporation Rate: N/D

pH: 3.11   (Butyl Acetate =1)

ENVIRONMENTAL DATA:——————————————————

SARA Reportability: NO   WHMIS Percentage: N/A

    Report as cas #: N/A   Subpart Z Status: N

    Reportable %: N/A   Clean Air Act: N

Sect. 313 Reportability: NO   Carcinogenity:

    Report as cas #: N/A   NTP: N, IARC: N

    Reportable %: N/A   OSHA: N

    RECRA Waste #: N/A   RECRA Reportable Qty.: N/A

========== ==============================

SECTION III: HAZARDOUS INGREDIENTS

========== ==============================

HAZARDOUS INGREDIENTS

???M: None

LD50 =	ACGIH =
TLV =	PEL =
STEL =	NIOSH =
IDLH =	RTECS =
CAS# =	NONE
Hazard: NONE	** ???

========== ==============================

SECTION IV: FIRE & EXPLOSION HAZARDS

========== ==============================

*   ??? ashpoint: NONE
*   Flammable Limits by Air: N/D
*   FIRE EXTINGUISHING METHOD:

    Water Spray

    Material Itself Is Not Combustible. If Involved In A Fire, Choose

       Extinguishing Agent Most Suitable For Type Of

    Surrounding Fire.

    Water

*   FIRE FIGHTING PROTECTION:

Run-Off May Contain Hazardous Materials And Should Be
Controlled If Necessary.

Wear Bunker Gear

Wear SCBA (Self Contained Breathing Apparatus)

* FIRE AND EXPLOSION HAZARDS:

Violent Rupture Of Containers Due To Heat Is Possible at
temperatures above 100'F.

========= ==========================

SECTION V: REACTIVITY DATA

========= ==========================

* STABILITY: Stable
* Conditions To Avoid:

Contamination From Any Outside Source

Do Not Mix With Bases, Caustics, Or Alkalies.

Keep Away From Fire, Open Flame, Or Any Heat Source.

Do Not Mix With Strong Oxidizers; Chlorines, Nitrites, Or
Peroxides.

* BYPRODUCTS OF DECOMPOSITION: (TOXIC VAPORS
FORMED & ETC.) Oxides Of Nitrogen Formed.

* HAZARDOUS POLYMERIZATON: Will Not Occur.

========= ==========================

SECTION VI: SPILL OR LEAK PROCEDURES

========= ==========================

CONSULT SECTION VII FOR PROPER SAFETY EQUIPMENT

DIKE SPILL AND PROTECT SEWER AND WATER INTAKE

VENTILATE AREA, MONITOR AIR FOR ACCUMULATION
OF HAZARDOUS VAPORS

NOTIFY ALL PROPER AUTHORITIES IF REQUIRED IN CASE
OF SPILL

FOLLOW ENVIRONMENTAL REGULATIONS

Carefully Neutralize With Weak Alkali Solution.

Use "SASCO ACID HANDLER" To Safely Solidify And Neutralize Spills Of This Product.

Rinse Residue Down The Drain With Plenty Of Water.

Use Large Amounts Of Water To Dilute Product Prior To Discharge.

WASTE DISPOSAL:

Follow Local, State, And Federal Disposal Regulations.

Consult S & S Co. For Further Information

Can Be Neutralized, As Noted, And Disposed Of In Accordance With Local, State, And Federal Regulations.

========== ========================

SECTION VII: SPECIAL PROTECTION INFORMATION

========== ========================

PROTECTION LEVELS SHOULD BE INCREASED ACCORDING TO THE SIZE OF THE SPILL. UNCOATED TYVEK SHOULD NEVER BE USED FOR CHEMICALS.

RESPIRATORY:

USE OF RESPIRATOR FOR FORMALDEHYDE MAY BE NECESSARY

DO TO SIZE OF SPILL

None Needed For Normal Use.

**   ??? IN CONTACT:

Latex/Rubber Gloves

**   EYE CONTACT:

Chemical Splash Goggles

**   VENTILATION:

Adequate For Work Area.

Maintain Levels Below TLV.

========== ========================

SECTION VIII: SPECIAL PRECAUTIONS
(HANDLING AND STORAGE)

========== ========================

** SPECIAL PRECAUTIONS:

Do Not Transfer To Containers Not Properly Labeled For This
Product.

Do Not Contaminate With Dirty Equipment.

** Use This Product At Room Temperature. Do Not Heat.

** OTHER PRECAUTIONS:

KEEP OUT OF REACH OF CHILDREN. FOR
INDUSTRIAL AND COMMERCIAL USE ONLY.

========== ========================

SECTION IX: HEALTH HAZARD DATA/ROUTES OF ENTRY

========== ========================

** TLV AND SOURCE: N/D

** ACUTE EFFECTS OF OVEREXPOSURE

** ???GESTION SYMPTOMS:

May Cause Diarrhea/Intestinal Distention/Cramps.

May Cause Irritation And Burning Of Membranes In Mouth &
Throat

May Cause Stomach Pain And Possible Ulceration.

** SKIN ABSORPTION And/Or SKIN CONTACT:

Repeated Or Prolonged Contact Causes Drying, Brittleness,
Cracking, And Irritation Of The Skin.

Repeated Or Prolonged Contact May Cause Drying, Brittleness,
Cracking, And Irritation Of The Skin. Prolonged Contact May
Cause Severe Burns On Sensitive Skin.

* RESPIRATORY:

Breathing Product Dust Or Mist May Irritate Respiratory Tract.

* EYE CONTACT:

 May Cause Inflammation Of The Conjunctives.

 May Cause Redness/Blurred Vision/Tearing/Burning.

* CHRONIC EFFECTS OF OVEREXPOSURE:

========== =========================

 ******* EMERGENCY AND FIRST AID PROCEDURES *******

========== =========================

* INGESTION:

 If Vomiting Occurs Spontaneously, Hold Head Lower Than Hips To Prevent Aspiration.

 Rinse Mouth Out And Spit. Do Not Swallow!

 Do Not Induce Vomiting. Drink Water Or Milk. Continue Sipping Fluids Until Medical Help Is Obtained.

 Keep Quiet And Treat For Shock. Do Not Speak Except To Assist In First Aid.

More Terminology

Hypo: A Greek element meaning under, lower, below, diminished

1. Hypodermic   under the skin
2. Hypofunction   abnormally diminished functions
3. Hypogene   formed under the earth's surface
4. Hypoglycemia   abnormally low blood sugar level
5. Hypokinesia   having diminished motor functions
6. Hyponoia   diminished function of thought
7. Hypoysis   to grow beneath
8. Hypotension   low blood pressure
9. Hypothermia   the artificial slowing of body temperature
10. Hypoxia   oxygen deficiency to body tissues

Safety for Health-Care Careers

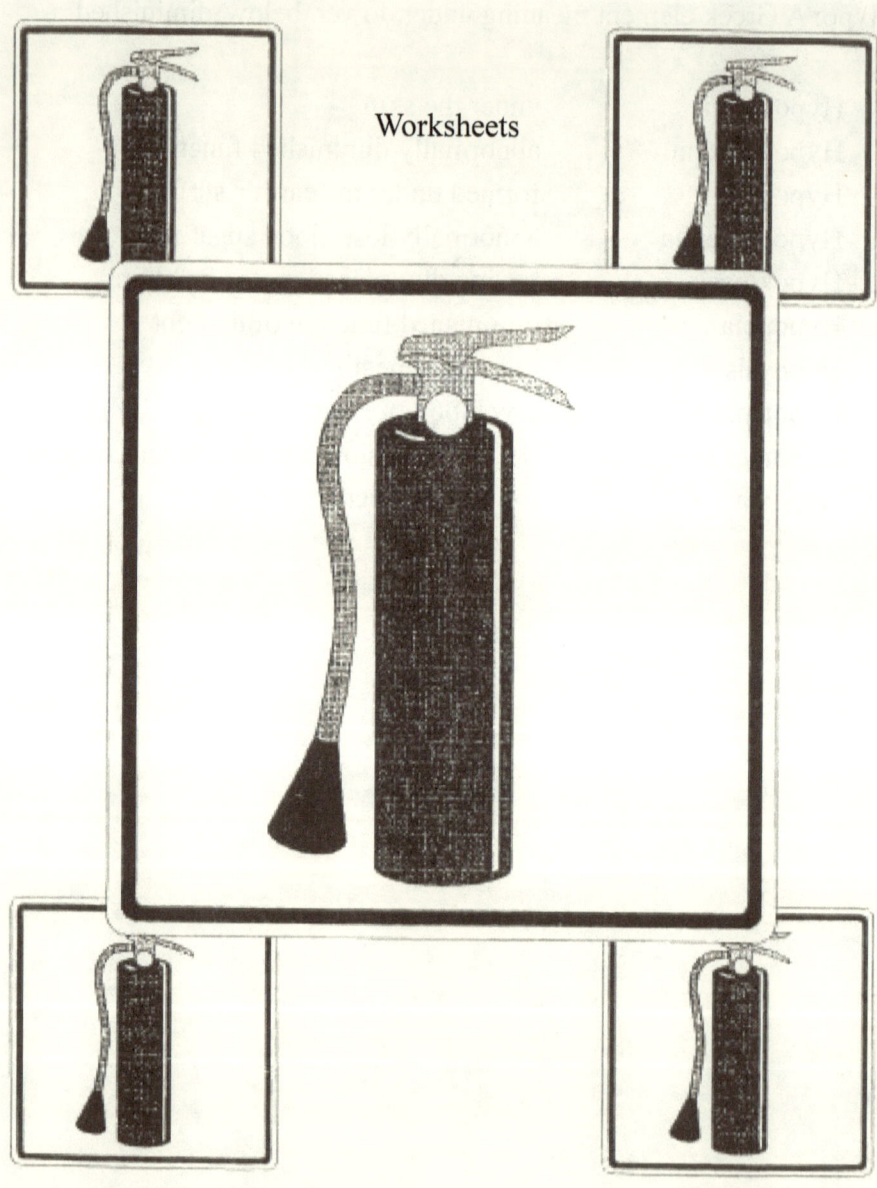

Worksheets

Student _____ Completion date _____ - _____ - _____

Instructor's signature for completion

Safety Review Worksheet

Directions: Write true (T) or false (F) in the slots provided.

1. ____ Incident reports should be written at the end of your shift.
2. ____ Pathogens help prevent infections.
3. ____ MSDS is a very dangerous chemical.
4. ____ An incident report cannot be used in a lawsuit because it contains confidential information.
5. ____ Oxygen is highly combustible.
6. ____ Pathogens cause an infection.
7. ____ Falls can be prevented by making sure there is adequate lighting.
8. ____ The spread of infection is not a health hazard in health-care facilities.
9. ____ Handrails provide support when walking up or down the stairs.
10. ____ You check glass and plastic equipment for damage prior to using.
11. ____ Smoking is allowed where oxygen is being used if there is not a No Smoking sign.
12. ____ You should not close doors or windows when a fire is in progress.
13. ____ A sudden event in which many are killed and injured and property is damaged is called a disaster.
14. ____ Universal precautions were issued by the CDC in 1887.
15. ____ Universal precautions were issued because of the Black Plague.
16. ____ RACE is an acronym for React, Activate, Combustion, Escape.
17. ____ Universal precautions were established by OSHA.
18. ____ Hand washing helps prevent the spread of pathogens.
19. ____ There are seven categories of infection precautions.
20. ____ Enteric precautions help prevent airborne infections.

21. ____ Report spilled liquids to your supervisor, then wipe the area dry.
22. ____ There are three basic types of fire extinguishers.
23. ____ There are three elements required to start a fire.
24. ____ RACE tells how a chemical should be used, stored, and removed.
25. ____ Malfunctioning equipment can cause electrical shock.
26. ____ A triage disaster plan describes the priority for action in the event of a disaster.
27. ____ A document that tells how a chemical is to be used, stored, and removed is called an MSDS.
28. ____ Each employee is responsible for knowing the evacuation exits at his or her workplace.
29. ____ C-rated fire extinguishers are used to stop electrical fires.
30. ____ To prevent fires, provide ashtrays in areas where smoking is allowed.
31. ____ Some pathogens are airborne.
32. ____ AFB precautions prevent the spread of pathogens through feces.
33. ____ You should tape any exposed electrical wiring before your supervisor observes it.
34. ____ Most safety rules are common sense.
35. ____ In the event of a disaster, you are responsible not only for yourself but also for patients, coworkers, and visitors.

Directions: Fill in the blanks with the appropriate response.

36. Do not smoke when _____ is in use.
37. Use a type _____ fire extinguisher to extinguish oil-based fires.
38. A/an _____ disaster plan tells the priority for action in a disaster situation.
39. The first step in a disaster plan is to _____ patients, visitors, and injured victims from danger.
40. To remove, activate, contain, and extinguish a fire is referred to by the acronym _____.

41. A/an _____ report is used to report unusual occurrences or accidents.

42. MSDS stands for _____ safety data sheet.

43. Infections are caused by microorganisms called _____.

44. Procedures to prevent infections caused by contact with blood, body fluids, or body substances are called _____ precautions.

45. Extra oxygen helps _____ when heat and fuel are available.

46. A No Smoking: _____ in Use sign should be posted in areas using oxygen.

47. You should be _____ conscious at all times.

48. Fire safety involves two primary areas: prevention and _____.

49. _____-rated extinguishers can stop wood, liquid, and electrical fires.

50. When working with chemicals, read the _____ before using them.

51. The _____ contains information about a chemical such as its properties, which is helpful in the event of fire or exposure.

52. The three elements for fire are heat, oxygen, and _____.

53. A/an _____-pronged grounding plug is used to prevent electrical shock.

54. Your hands must be _____ when using electrical equipment.

55. All incident reports should contain the _____ Ws.

56. Incident reports must be accurate because they may be used in a/an _____ suit.

57. Evacuation plans should be _____ throughout each health-care facility.

58. The CDC enacted universal precautions in the year _____.

59. The CDC acknowledged _____ areas of precaution.

60. The _____ area of precaution is designed to prevent pathogen spread through feces.

Directions: Circle the letter of the *best* answer.

61. In the event of a fire, you should do all except _____.

    a. catch the nearest elevator out
    b. sound the fire alarm
    c. call the switchboard operator
    d. do not panic

62. Electrical fires are extinguished by _____-rated fire extinguishers.

    e. A
    f. B
    g. C
    h. ABC

63. It takes _____ things to start a fire.

    a. 3
    b. 2
    c. 4
    d. none of the above

64. Oxygen is all of the terms below except _____.

    a. liquid
    b. clear
    c. combustible
    d. all around us

65. Spills should be cleaned _____.

    a. after reporting them to the appropriate supervisor
    b. after writing an incident report
    c. by the janitor
    d. immediately

66. All the terms below are areas of universal precautions except _____.

    a. AFB
    b. enteric
    c. generic
    d. strict

67. In the event of a disaster, _____.

    a. initiate triage procedures
    b. run for help
    c. call your supervisor for help
    d. none of the above

68. Oxygen should not be used _____.

    a. while smoking
    b. near fire
    c. near heat
    d. all of the above

69. Universal precautions _____.

    a. are used only in California
    b. deal only with airborne pathogens
    c. warns us of universally contracted diseases
    d. require gowns, masks, and gloves

70. In a triage disaster plan, _____.

    a. women and children are cared for first
    b. those with clogged airways are cared for first
    c. treat those with severe bleeding first
    d. treat those in shock first

71. Each health-care facility should have_____.

   a. a copy of the universal precautions posted
   b. an evacuation escape plan posted
   c. an established triage disaster plan
   d. all of the above

72. General safety rules include_____.

   a. being safety conscious at all times
   b. acknowledging safety and warning signs
   c. using handrails
   d. all of the above

73. Pathogens enter the body through all except the_____.

   a. reproductive system
   b. respiratory system
   c. integumentary system
   d. all of the above

74. Enteric precautions prevent the _____.

   a. patient from coming in contact with pathogens
   b. spread of pathogens found in wounds
   c. spread of pathogens through fecal materials
   d. spread of pathogens through the air

75. MSDS refers to_____.

   a. material safety data sheet
   b. management safety data sheet
   c. malicious safety data sheet
   d. none of the above

Directions: Match the definition to the letter of the word it best describes.

76. A microorganism that causes infections.

a. CDC

77. Occurs when heat, fuel, and oxygen are combined.

b. respiratory

78. Describes the properties and safe use of a chemical.

c. incident report

79. A procedure for fighting fires.

d. shock

80. A form for documenting unusual events.

e. triage disaster plan

81. An organization that enacted universal precautions.

f. pathogen

82. A procedure for prioritizing when a disaster occurs.

g. RACE

83. A body system that allows pathogens to enter the body through the air.

h. combustion

84. An element required for the starting of a fire.

i. MSDS

85. Three-pronged electric plugs are used to prevent_____.

j. fuel

Directions: Define each term below.

86. MSDS

_____

_____

_____

87. Oxygen_____

_____

_____

88. Triage

_____

_____

_____

89. Incident

_____

_____

_____

90. 5 Ws

_____

_____

_____

91. Disaster

_____

_____

_____

92. Evacuation

93. Pathogens

94. RACE

95. Infection

Sabrina Hutton Edmond

Answer Sheet for Safety

Student _____ Date _____ Instructor Initial _____

1. _____
2. _____
3. _____
4. _____
5. _____
6. _____
7. _____
8. _____
9. _____
10. _____
11. _____
12. _____
13. _____
14. _____
15. _____
16. _____
17. _____
18. _____
19. _____
20. _____
21. _____
22. _____
23. _____

24. _____
25. _____
26. _____
27. _____
28. _____
29. _____
30. _____
31. _____
32. _____
33. _____
34. _____
35. _____
36. _____
37. _____
38. _____
39. _____
40. _____
41. _____
42. _____
43. _____
44. _____
45. _____
46. _____
47. _____
48. _____
49. _____

50. _____

51. _____

52. _____

53. _____

54. _____

55. _____

56. _____

57. _____

58. _____

59. _____

60. _____

61. a b c d

62. a b c d

63. a b c d

64. a b c d

65. a b c d

66. a b c d

67. a b c d

68. a b c d

69. a b c d

70. a b c d

71. a b c d

72. a b c d

73. a b c d

74. a b c d

75. a b c d

76. _____
77. _____
78. _____
79. _____
80. _____
81. _____
82. _____
83. _____
84. _____
85. _____

86 to 95: Define on a sheet of paper on the next page.

Analysis

Problems   95
Number incorrect   _____
Number correct   _____
Percent correct   %

Introduction to Health Science

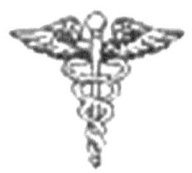

Unit 4

Nutrition

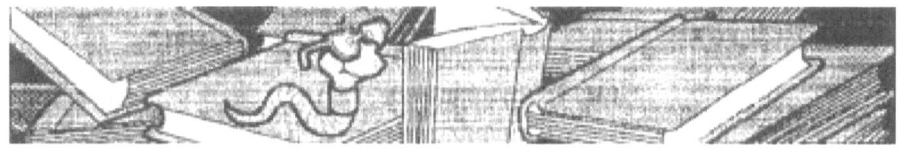

Eat a Variety of Foods

The body needs nutrients in order to perform properly and to fight off disease. Nutrients provide the body with fibers, vitamins, minerals, and fat. To assure that your body is receiving the proper amount of nutrients, it is important for you to eat a balanced diet. No one food group or vitamin-and-mineral supplement will provide your body with all its dietary needs. A good diet will include daily servings from each of the four food groups: fruits and vegetables, proteins, grains, and dairy foods.

Fruits and vegetables provide the body with specific vitamins and minerals. These vitamins include vitamins A, B, C, E, and K. These vitamins can help the body grow; increase vision; promote healthy skin; release energy from food within the body's cells; promote strong teeth, gums, and walls in blood vessels; help in the proper formation of connective tissues; prevent oxidation of certain fatty substances in the body; and provide for normal clotting of blood.

Protein foods help the body heal itself and fight diseases and infections. Most foods that contain protein also have vitamins and minerals. Protein helps provide the body with energy.

The human body is an amazing machine. Hundreds of organs work together every second to assure its ability to function properly. To continue to function properly, the body needs proper care. You can protect your body by developing good health habits and obtaining knowledge of how to keep the body functioning properly. You can harm your body by upsetting the perfect balance that nature has given it. Smoking, drug abuse, lack of rest, unsafe sex, poor nutrition, lack of exercise, and various other unhealthy habits can contribute to poor health and early death.

Learning about health should be a part of everyone's education. Advances in health science have helped *alleviate* some illnesses, provide cures for some, and make others more bearable. Vaccination programs and antibiotic drugs are just a few of the medical advances that have helped make us healthier. In this course, our major goal will be to make you more conscious of health-related decisions and give you a brief introduction to the body and ways to help you maintain its delicate balance.

Excessive weight may also cause psychological problems due to low self-esteem, teasing by others, discrimination in the workplace, and other forms of weight discrimination.

Avoid Too Much Fat and Cholesterol

Cholesterol and saturated fats have been, in recent years, attributed to breast, prostate, colon, and rectum cancers. Because most overweight people consume diets high in fats and cholesterol, obesity has been directly attributed to heart disease, increased blood pressure, heart attack, coronary heart disease, coronary blockage, and stroke. Science contends that a diet low in saturated fats and cholesterol may reduce many cancer risks, obesity, and ailments associated with obesity. Although some fat is essential for the body and some cholesterol—called good cholesterol or high-density lipoprotein (HDL)—is an important part of the membranes of each cell in the human body, most physicians and nutritionist recommend a diet low in fat and cholesterol. Many scientific studies have shown that low fat and cholesterol levels in the blood will significantly reduce heart attacks.

Eat Foods with Adequate Starch and Fiber

Most health experts and nutritionists recommend that we increase our intake of starch and fiber in our diets. Starch helps the body increase its energy, and high-fiber diets may reduce the risk of colon and rectal cancers. Fiber and starch sources include vegetables, potatoes, whole-grain breads, whole-grain cereals, dry peas, and beans. A diet high in fiber and starch also increases your B-vitamin intake and is a good source for calcium (bone-and-tooth strengthener).

Avoid Alcoholic Beverages or Drink in Moderation

Drinking alcoholic beverages can lead to many minor and major health problems when it is done in excess. Alcoholic beverages are high in calories and low in vitamins and minerals. It has been suggested in some studies that moderate consumption of wine (two or fewer drinks each day) may be helpful; however, most doctors and scientists maintain that *abstinence* from alcoholic beverages would be preferable. Excessive or abusive consumption of alcoholic beverages can lead to cancer of the mouth, throat, esophagus, bladder, and liver. It can also lead to birth defects and/or miscarriages. The use of alcoholic beverages, along with smoking, is considered to be especially risky and harmful to the body.

Today, most nutritionists, doctors, and scientists believe that consuming a well-balanced diet, along with exercise, will help maintain a healthy body and mind. Being nutrition conscious will help prevent disease, cure disease, and increase life expectancy. Proper nutrition can help determine if you are in the high-risk group or the low-risk group for contracting certain diseases. This is considered to be especially true with cancer.

Maintaining a nutritious diet does not require you to eat only foods or dishes that you do not enjoy; it only requires that you be conscious of your diet and begin to choose more of some foods and less of others.

The following chart is designed to help you select nutritious items for your breakfast, lunch, and dinner. It only suggests broad food areas and is designed to help you use a variety of foods in your diet. Remember, a good diet will include proteins, starches, fruits, and vegetables in each meal. Choosing from these four areas will also provide the fats, minerals, vitamins, and fibers needed to keep the body functioning properly. Use the "Choose Often" list as much as possible, use the "Choose Moderately" list sparingly, and try to avoid those in the "Avoid" list—although it is OK to use them occasionally.

4. Sanitize all food preparation areas.
5. Wash your hands before handling foods to be prepared.

The three most common food poisons are caused by staphylococcus, salmonella, and botulinum. All are potentially lethal; however, with proper handling, sanitation, and cooking of food, they can be readily destroyed. Freezing foods does not kill *microbes* (disease-causing microscopic organism). It only prevents or slows down the growth of microbes. Food-poisoning organisms can grow in foods when their temperatures exceed 45° to 50°F (7° to 10°C). Frozen foods should be refrigerated at or below 0°F (-18°C).

Carbohydrates are starches that furnish the body with energy and help strengthen our immune systems. Grains are our major source for carbohydrates.

Dairy foods provide protein, vitamins, calcium, and other minerals. Dairy products promote strong teeth and bones. These products have been known to prevent and/or slow down the onset of osteoarthritis and other joint diseases in women and men. Dairy products are essential for the growth of teeth and bones in young children.

Diseases such as scurvy, beriberi, xerophthalmia, night blindness, pellagra, rickets, and pernicious anemia can all be prevented and/or cured when the diet includes the foods with the specific vitamins whose absence causes the diseases to develop.

Maintain Desirable Weight

Excessive weight gain or *obesity* has been attributed to many illnesses including heart disease, bone disease, high blood pressure, diabetes, and certain types of cancer. Obesity can be prevented or corrected by maintaining a proper diet and starting a daily exercise routine.

What's in a Serving?

To help you plan healthy meals, we list below some examples of what constitutes a serving size for each of the Food Guide Pyramid groups. We include tips from Kaiser Permanente nutritionists and indicate the number of daily servings for each group.

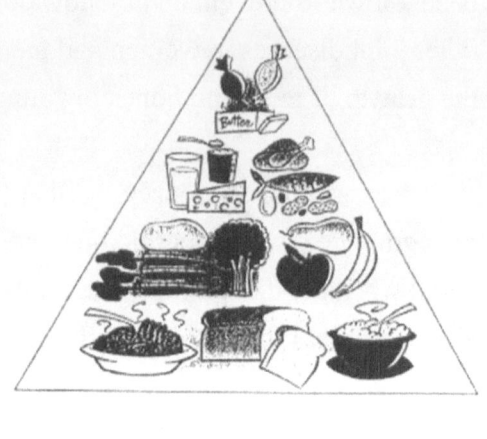

Bread Group (6 to 11 servings)

1 slice of bread (or about 1 ounce)
½ cup cooked rice, pasta, or other grains
½ cup cooked cereal
1 ounce cold cereal

Loudon says it's OK to eat more than one serving of cereal at a time because the recommendation from the bread group is 6 to 11 servings per day.

Both Loudon and Voight say you should read food labels to become aware of the serving sizes and nutritional content you're getting.

Vegetable Group (3 to 6 servings)

½ cup cooked or chopped raw vegetables
1 cup raw green leafy vegetables
¾ cup vegetable juice

Most vegetables are so low in calories and contain so many nutrients that eating more than the recommended number of servings is health??? four nutritionists say that most Americans don't eat enough vegetables.

Fruit Group (2 to 4 servings)

1 medium-size piece of fruit
¼ cantaloupe or other small melon
½ cup canned fruit, drained or packed in its own juice
¾ cup juice
¼ cup dried fruit

As with vegetables, most Americans don't eat enough fruit, so it may be better to err in the direction of too much. Sparks says that while fruit juice is generally a healthy beverage choice, in order to get the benefit of fiber, it's always better to eat fruit than to drink it.

Meat Group (2 to 3 servings)

2 ½ to 3 ounces cooked lean meat or poultry (without skin)

2 ½ to 3 ounces cooked fish
½ cup cooked beans; 1 egg; 2 tablespoons peanut butter (all equal 1 ounce of meat)

Voight offers this rule to help visualize a Food Guide Pyramid—size serving of meat: "You have two hands, so you'll know: each of your two daily servings of meat should be about the size of your palm and the thickness of your baby finger."

Dairy Group (2 to 3 servings)

1 cup low-fat or skim milk
1 cup low or nonfat yogurt
1 ½ ounces low-fat or fat-free cheese (about 1 ½ inches square)

Loudon tells people to grate their cheese because it looks like more. She adds that low-fat cheese is a healthy choice—it has to comply with the government definition for low-fat foods, which means no more than 3 grams of fat per serving.

Sparks says that many people don't get enough calcium because they don't want the fat that comes with dairy products. In addition to low-fat dairy products, try calcium-fortified orange juice.

Fats, Oils, and Sweets Group (use sparingly)

Your daily intake of fats should equal less than 30 percent of your daily calorie intake. Sparks says your daily intake of sugar should equal no more than 10 percent of your daily calorie intake.

Loudon offers this salad-bar survival tip: get the dressing on the side and dip your fork in the dressing first and then in your salad—you'll eat much less fat without sacrificing much of the flavor.

Introduction to Body Systems

The human body in this phase will be divided into ten body systems. All living things begin with chemicals. These chemicals combine to form complex substances that form living cells. Cells combine and form tissues. Tissues combine to form organs. When a group of organs work together for the same general purpose, they form body systems.

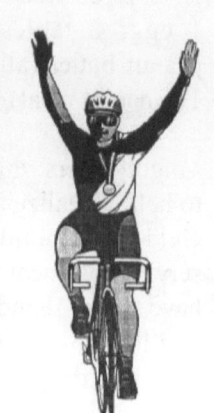

In this phase, you will be given a brief description of each of the ten body systems. If you would like a more thorough understanding of any or all the body systems discussed in this chapter, information can be obtained from any good anatomy book or from a good encyclopedia. As stated earlier, this course is not designed to substitute for an anatomy or any other science class; this chapter is merely designed to give you a general overview of the human anatomy and its ten body systems.

The Skeletal System

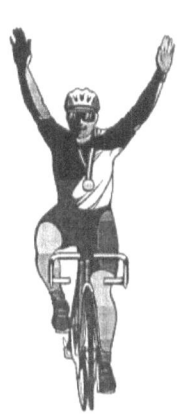

A car has many moving parts and accessories. These parts, when working together properly, provide for smooth starting, moving, and stopping. All the moving parts and accessories on an automobile are held together or attached to the automobile frame. The human body, like an automobile, is held together by a frame. We call this frame the skeletal system. It is the basic framework of the body. The skeletal system consists collectively of over two hundred bones and joints.

Bones are the framework of the skeletal system. Bones are composed of tissues that contain blood vessels and nerves. Bones connect to other bones at points called joints. Joints are connected by either cartilage or ligaments. Joints can be categorized by the amount of movement they allow. Fibrous joints are immovable. Cartilaginous joints are slightly movable. Synovial joints are freely movable.

Bones and joints are the basis of the skeletal system. The skeletal system serves six basic functions:

1. Provides framework for the body
2. Protects other body organs
3. Serves as a lever for movement
4. Serves as a storehouse for calcium
5. Produces blood cells
6. Allows body movement

As stated earlier, the skeleton consists of over two hundred bones and joints. In this lesson, we will divide the skeletal system into four sections: cranial section, trunk, upper limbs, and lower limbs.

The cranial skeleton consists of the skull, upper and lower jawbones, and neck bones. The main function of the bones and joints in the cranial section is to protect the brain and eyes. It also serves to provide movement of the skull.

The trunk section is divided into two parts: the upper trunk and the lower trunk. The upper trunk section includes the rib cage that protects the heart and lungs, the pelvic bones that support the weight of the upper body and that allow for its movement, the shoulder bones that connect the arms to the upper body and allow for arm movement, and the spinal bones that protect the spinal cord and provide the main support for the body and allow the upper body to bend and twist. The lower section of the trunk protects the liver, kidney, reproductive system, stomach, and pancreas.

The upper limbs are the section of the skeletal system that consists of the arm bones, hand bones, and wrist bones. These bone structures allow complicated movement such as grasping and writing. The upper limbs also allow for touch.

The lower limbs are the section of the skeletal system that supports the weight of the upper body and allows for running, jumping, and walking. The lower limbs include the leg bones, feet bones, ankle bones, toe bones, and kneecaps. These bone structures also help balance the body.

The Muscular System

Muscles can be seen as the body's movers. There are more than 650 individual muscles in the human body. These muscles work in pairs by pulling. Muscles compose nearly 40% of our body weight.

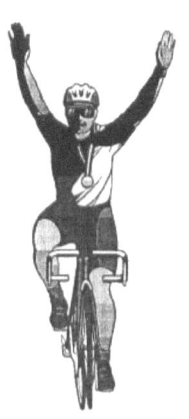

The muscle is a tissue made up of thin fibers that work together to allow body movement. Each muscle fiber is connected to a nerve. Nerves receive their instructions from the brain (a message center) and relay the information to the muscles. Nerves relay messages from the brain to the muscles that tell the muscles when and how much to contract.

The body has three kinds of muscle tissues. Skeletal muscles are voluntary muscles (controlled by will). This muscle tissue controls body movement. Smooth muscles are involuntary (not controlled by will). Arteries are examples of smooth muscle tissues. The cardiac muscle is the strongest muscle in the body. The cardiac muscle tissue is involuntary and works without conscious commands from the mind. Cardiac muscles pump blood to the body's circulatory system. All muscles pull. The muscles pull because of their ability to make themselves shorter and fatter. This is called contraction. Every bone or organ in the body that moves, pumps, or pushes is controlled by a pair of muscles. This pair of muscles is called antagonistic muscles because they work against each other. When one muscle pulls, the other relaxes. The muscle that moves is called the prime mover. The muscle that relaxes or produces an opposite movement is called the antagonist.

The Digestive System

The digestive system consists basically of the alimentary canal—one continuous tube that connects the mouth and all the organs between it to the anal opening. As you recall, cells form organs, and a group of organs working together to perform a specific function form body organ systems. The digestive system is a body organ system. The digestive system is composed of seven basic organs: mouth, esophagus, stomach, small intestine, large intestine, liver, and the pancreas.

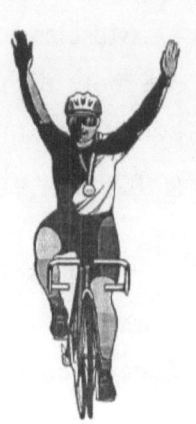

The mouth is used to prepare food for digestion. In the mouth, food is ground and mixed with saliva—a solution that contains approximately 95% water; the enzyme amylase, which begins to break down starches; and mucus, which lubricates the food.

The esophagus is a tubelike organ that carries food from the mouth to the stomach by use of involuntary contractions of its walls.

The stomach is the organ in the digestive system that uses pepsin, an enzyme that helps break down protein. Hydrochloric acid is secreted to activate the pepsin, to dissolve minerals, and to kill bacteria that enters the stomach with food. Because the stomach secretes acid, it must also secrete mucus to neutralize the acids to protect the stomach's lining.

The small intestine absorbs the water from the waste and by-products of the stomach. Once the water is absorbed, it leaves undigested materials in a solid state. The undigested materials pass through the large intestine and out of the anal opening.

The pancreas is a body organ that secretes enzymes into the stomach to break down proteins, starches, and fats.

The liver is a body organ that secretes bile from the gall bladder into the stomach. Bile, an alkalized liquid, breaks up large fat globules into smaller droplets to be passed to the large intestine. Once food has been digested, its nutrients pass through the small intestine and into the bloodstream. Remaining undigested food is then passed to the large intestine, where it is stored and eliminated from the body. The large intestine is also responsible for reabsorbing water in the digestive tract and returning it back to the body, preventing dehydration. When the large intestine eliminates undigested food through the anal canal and completes the reabsorption of water, the digestive cycle is completed.

The Circulatory System

The circulatory system is responsible for sending nutrients and oxygen to the body's cells and carrying away the cells' by-products and waste materials. It is actually a one-way transport system that carries blood throughout the body.

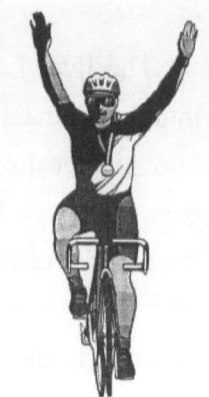

The center of the circulatory system is the heart. The heart pumps hemoglobin (blood) into the blood vessels. Hemoglobin is composed of plasma, the liquid portion; red blood cells, cells that carry oxygen; white blood cells, cells that fight infection and disease; and thrombocytes, cell fragments that help in coagulation (blood clotting) to seal wounds.

The heart is a muscle that consists of four chambers: the right atrium, left atrium, right ventricle, and left ventricle. The right ventricle receives deoxygenated blood from the right atrium, and the right ventricle then pumps the deoxygenated blood into the lungs, where it is oxygenated. Oxygenated blood then flows to the left atrium. The oxygenated blood from the left atrium is then pumped into the left ventricle. From the left ventricle, oxygenated blood flows to all of the body's cells. Once deoxygenated, the blood is pumped to the right atrium. When the deoxygenated blood reaches the right atrium, the cycle starts over.

The heart uses blood vessels to help it perform its work. The heart pumps hemoglobin into these vessels. There are three kinds of blood vessels: arteries, capillaries, and veins.

Arteries are blood vessels that carry blood away from the heart. Capillaries are very small vessels that branch from the arteries. The capillaries supply nutrients and oxygen in the blood to the cells. Veins are the smallest blood vessels; they transport blood back to the heart, carbon dioxide to the lungs, and waste products of the cells to the kidneys. The veins have very low pressure. Veins have flaps called valves that prevent blood from flowing backward and allow the blood to return back to the right atrium.

In conclusion, the circulatory system transports hemoglobin throughout the body by use of the heart, arteries, veins, and capillaries in order to perform various important body functions including the following:

1. Providing oxygen from the lungs to cells
2. Carrying carbon dioxide to the lungs
3. Absorbing nutrients and carrying them to the cells
4. Carrying waste products to be excreted from the body
5. Transporting hormones (chemical messengers that regulate cells)
6. Regulating body temperature
7. Helping maintain the fluid balance of the body
8. Defending the body against infection and disease

The Respiratory System

Your body's nutrients are converted to energy that is released to its cells. This process is called cellular respiration. When cellular respiration takes place, the cells take in oxygen and expel carbon dioxide along with small amounts of water called water vapor. Cellular respiration has three phases: ventilation, diffusion, and transport. These three phases are made possible by the body's respiratory system. The respiratory system is a system of cartilage, tubes, and muscles that form a 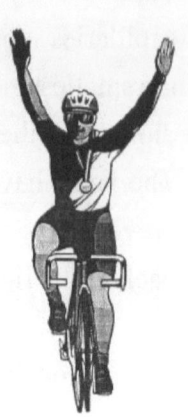 pathway for air to be brought to cells and their by-products released in the atmosphere.

The pharynx is a muscle that carries air into the respiratory tract along with performing digestive and other functions. The larynx is a tube consisting of cartilage and chambers, which receives air from the pharynx. The larynx serves in the production of speech due to the way air flows from the lungs around the vocal cords inside the larynx. The larynx also helps prevent food from mixing with the air in the remainder of the respiratory tract.

The trachea (windpipe) conducts air between the larynx and the lungs. The trachea is a tube consisting of a C-shaped cartilage that keeps it open and allows air to pass through.

The trachea divides into two branchlike areas called *bronchi*. The two bronchi enter the lungs and transport the air from the trachea to the lungs. The right bronchus is larger than the left bronchus. The blood vessels and nerves are also connected with each lung in its bronchus.

The right bronchus has an air sac called the alveoli. When the alveoli fills with air, it passes oxygen to the capillaries, where it is transported to all the body's cells.

The body has two lungs. Each lung is set inside an area called the thoracic or chest cavity. Each lung is covered by a closed sac called the pleura with the exception of the areas where the bronchi and blood vessels enter. It is in the lungs where respiration takes place. Again, respiration has three phases. The movement of air in and out of the lungs is known as ventilation. When oxygen is passed in the capillaries to the blood cells and carbon dioxide is passed out of the blood cells, diffusion takes place. The final phase is called transport. This takes place when oxygen is moved to the cells and carbon dioxide from the cells to the lungs. Transport is made possible by the circulation of blood through the respiratory system.

The diaphragm is a dome-shaped muscle that forms a partition between the lungs and the abdominal cavity. The diaphragm contracts and flattens to allow inhaling of air and relaxes to its dome shape to allow exhaling of carbon dioxide and water vapors.

The Nervous System

All the body systems work interdependently as one complete unit. The nervous system is the main coordinating system for the body. It responds to internal and external stimuli and allows the systems to adapt to new conditions to maintain homeostasis. Homeostasis is when a system is balanced and working properly. The nervous system receives messages from the other systems, analyzes it, and transmits instructions back to these systems.

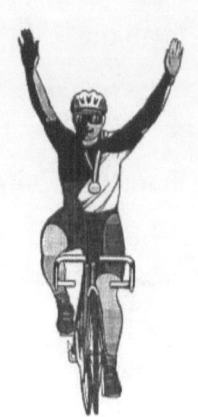

The nervous system is composed of the brain, spinal cord, and nerves. The brain and spinal cord form the central nervous system (CNS). The spinal cord has three basic functions: reflex activities that provide for rapid and automatic response to stimuli, conduction of sensory impulses to the brain, and conduction of motor impulses from the brain to the muscles or glands.

The spinal cord is a long, slender cord consisting of nerves that run down through the neck and back. Its function is to act as a message processing center for incoming messages from the peripheral nerves. Most messages carried to the spinal cord are relayed to the brain for its response. Other messages that require quick responses are handled directly by the spinal cord. When the spinal cord responds to the incoming messages, it causes reflex actions. Reflex actions are those responses that occur without conscious thought. If stuck by a needle, you would jump quickly—this is an example of a reflex action. Reflex actions generally protect us from dangers that might cause us great harm if we wait for the brain to respond.

The brain is located inside the cranial cavity. It is covered by three layers of connective tissue called meninges. Meninges contain membranes, fluids, and bones. Meninges also cover and protect the spinal cord. The average brain weighs about three pounds. It is a jellylike grayish-pink ball held in the cranial cavity, where a network of blood vessels supplies large quantities of oxygen and nutrients that it requires. The brain uses approximately 20% of the body's oxygen. The brain is the center of the body system. It governs speech; directs action; interprets external stimuli from impulses from the skin; receives and interprets auditory, olfactory, and visual impulses; regulates body movement and facial expressions; provides for thoughts, ideas, memory, and learning; and organizes information. All sensory impulses including those that control body temperature, water balance, sleep, appetite, thinking, breathing, fear, pleasure, conscious functions, and automatic functions are made possible by the brain. The brain also aids in the coordination of voluntary muscles and maintenance of muscle tone. The brain and spinal cord work together and are connected by the brain stem.

The brain stem controls vital body functions. These functions include beating of the heart, swallowing, and vomiting. The brain stem is made up of the midbrain, pons, and medulla oblongata. The pons connects the midbrain to the medulla; the medulla connects the brain to the spinal cord. The midbrain relays impulses to the eyes and ears. The pons connects the cerebellum to the rest of the nervous system. The medulla oblongata is the part of the brain stem that regulates vital body functions such as breathing, maintaining normal heartbeat rate and blood pressure, swallowing, vomiting, and blood flow.

The nerves act as sensory devices that send messages from the other body systems to the brain and receive instructions from the brain to send back to the other body systems by way of impulses. Afferent nerves have sensory fibers for conducting impulses or sending messages to the brain. Efferent nerves consist of motor fibers that move impulses away from the brain.

Nerves located in the cranial or spinal area make up the peripheral nervous system (PNS). These nerves are all located outside the CNS. The PNS also contains the autonomic nervous system. This system carries impulses from the CNS to the involuntary muscles, including the smooth muscles, cardiac muscles, and glands. The somatic nervous system is made up of nerves that control the actions of the skeletal muscles, which are under conscious control. The peripheral nervous system contains forty-three pairs of nerves.

The nervous system is the one body system that affects all the other body systems. It is probably the most complicated of all the systems, and it is definitely the least understood of all.

The Integumentary System

As you learned earlier, the body is a complex system of organs. These organs perform vital functions; however, none of them are protected from outside sources. The integumentary system is the body system designed to protect the other organs from harmful substances, bacteria, viruses, and ultraviolet rays. The integumentary system is composed of the skin, hair, nails, and sweat and oil glands.

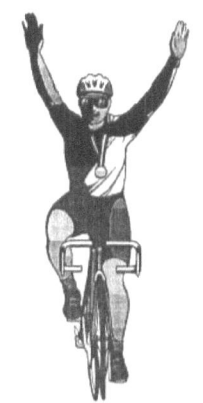

The skin is an elastic-like membrane (layer of tissue) that covers the body. The skin consists of two main layers: the epidermis and dermis. The epidermis is the surface layer of the skin. The epidermis contains no blood vessels; thus, it receives its nourishment from the capillaries in the underlying dermis. The epidermis constantly replenishes its dead cells with new cells, which are being continuously pushed upward to replace the dead cells. Melanin, a pigment that gives skin its color, is produced in the epidermis. The dermis consists of elastic connective tissue that contains muscles, nerves, capillaries, oil glands, and sweat glands. The dermis's primary function is to provide nourishment to the epidermis, regenerate cells for the dead skin of the epidermis, and supply keratin (a protein) to the epidermis.

The subcutaneous layer is located below the dermis. The subcutaneous layer connects the skin to the surface muscles. It consists of elastic and fibrous connective tissue and fat tissue. The fat serves as insulation and is also used to store reserved energy. The elastic fibers connect subcutaneous tissue with the dermis. Major blood vessels to the skin and many of the skin appendages such as nails, hair, sweat glands, and oil glands extend into the subcutaneous tissue. Nerves and nerve endings are routed throughout the subcutaneous layer.

The sebaceous glands are glands that secrete an oily substance called sebum, which helps keep the skin elastic. The sebaceous glands are important in the prevention of dry, splitting skin and in the lubrication of the hair.

The sweat glands or sudoriferous glands secrete water, mineral salt, and other substances in order to help cool down the body and regulate temperature. Each gland has an excretory tube that extends to the skin surface and opens at the pores. The sweat glands are located in the dermis. Some sweat glands secrete their substance in the armpits and groin area through the hair follicles due to emotional stress or sexual stimulation. The secretion from these glands is modified by bacteria and produces body odor. Wax in the ear canal and the tears around the eyelid are also secreted from glands similar to the sweat glands.

Hair and nails are two other appendages of the integumentary system. Hair can be found over most of the body although the amount of hair on each individual is different. Hair is not living; it is composed of a substance called keratin. Each hair develops from a follicle. New hair is formed from cells under the follicle. A thin band of involuntary muscle is attached to most hair follicles. These involuntary muscles cause the sebaceous glands to release sebum on the hair follicles.

Nails are protective structures found on the fingers and toes. Nails, like hair, are not living. Nails are also made of keratin; however, the keratin in nails is hard and produced by cells that start in the outside layer of the epidermis. New nail cells are formed continuously at the end of the nail and extend outwardly from the nail root.

In conclusion, the integumentary system provides a protective covering for the body systems. This covering includes the skin, nails, and hair. The system also includes glands that lubricate parts of the body and help regulate body temperature.

The Urinary System

The urinary or excretory system has four main components or organs. The urinary system's primary function is to excrete certain body wastes and excessive water from the body.

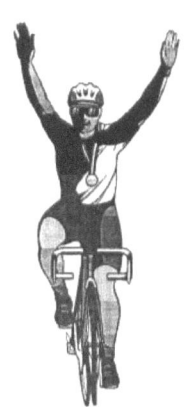

The human body has two kidneys. These two kidneys act as filters. The kidneys' major functions are to excrete waste products from cellular metabolism, excess salts, and toxic substances; to maintain water balance to acids and antacid balances; and to produce hormones to help regulate blood pressure and also prevent anemia (low red blood cell count). Urine is the liquid waste produced and excreted from the kidney after it filters the blood received from the renal arteries. Urine includes ammonia, urea, uric acid, excessive water, potassium, sodium, and other substances. The ureter is a tube that carries urine from the kidneys into the urinary bladder. The body has two ureters, one extending from each kidney. The ureters extend from the kidney to and through the urinary bladder. The ureters convey urine from the kidney to the urinary bladder by way of peristalsis (rhythmic muscle contraction) at frequent intervals.

The urinary bladder is a temporary reservoir used to hold urine. When the bladder is full of urine, it expels the urine into the urethra.

The urethra is a tube that extends from the bladder to the outside. The bladder empties its urine into the urethra. The urethra then expels the urine outside the body. The urethra is not the same in both men and women. In men, the urethra is longer than that of women, and it is also part of the male reproductive system. The male urethra carries semen during ejaculation and urine on other occasions. The male urethra passes through the prostate gland and is joined by two ducts carrying male sex cells. These cells then flow outside the body by way of the penis. In the female, the urethra serves one function—the removal of urine from the bladder.

The Endocrine System

The endocrine system consists of organs that produce hormones. Hormones are chemical messengers that help regulate body functions. Hormones are secreted by the endocrine glands. The endocrine system and nervous systems are the two main systems that control and coordinate other systems of the body.

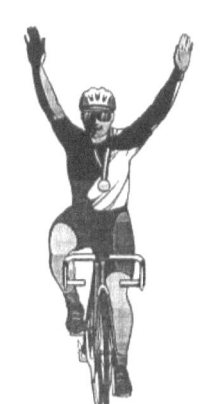

Hormones are released into tissue fluid and the bloodstream, where they are carried to other parts of the body. There are two kinds of hormones. Protein hormones make up most of the body's hormones. Steroid hormones regulate the adrenal cortex and the sex glands. All other hormones are protein. The endocrine system can be divided into six main gland groups.

The thyroid glands are the largest of the endocrine glands. The main hormone produced in the thyroid gland is thyroxine. Thyroxine, along with other growth hormones, promotes normal growth. Calcitonin is another hormone secreted by the thyroid gland and acts to decrease the amount of calcium in the bloodstream. The parathyroid glands secrete the hormone parathyroid hormone (PTH); it acts to promote the release of calcium from the bone tissue into the bloodstream and also controls the amount of phosphorous in the body.

The adrenal glands are divided into two parts. One is the adrenal medulla (inner portion). One hormone produced in the adrenal medulla is epinephrine. Epinephrine acts as a neurotransmitter. Norepinephrine—another hormone produced by the adrenal medulla glands—regulates blood pressure, converts glycogen to glucose for energy, increases the heart rate, increases the metabolic rate of body cells, and dilates the bronchiolus.

The adrenal cortex is the other part of the adrenal glands. The adrenal cortex glands secrete two main hormones. Glucocorticoids are hormones that suppress inflammatory responses. Mineralocorticoids regulate the body's electrolyte balance by controlling the reabsorption of sodium and the secretion of potassium by the kidneys.

The pancreas secretes the hormones glucagon and insulin. These hormones work together to regulate the amount of glucose in the cells of all body organs except the brain. The sex glands produce hormones that are essential in the development of sexual characteristics. Testosterone is the main male sex hormone; it promotes voice deepening, facial and body hair, voice tone. Progesterone is a female hormone. It promotes normal pregnancy and prepares the female uterine for implantation of fertilized ovum (female sex cells).

The pituitary glands are controlled by the nervous system. They in turn help regulate other body systems. The pituitary glands release hormones that affect the working of other glands. Their hormones stimulate the thyroid glands, adrenal cortex glands, and the sex glands. The pituitary glands also produce antidiuretic hormones that promote the reabsorption of water in the kidneys.

The Reproductive System

The reproductive system is essential for the perpetuation of the human species. Reproduction in humans is sexual; this means that it takes a male and female to perpetuate other males and females. Both the male and female have cells that specialize in sex. In the male, these cells are called spermatozoa. In the female, these cells are called ova. These sex cells, referred to as germ cells, contain half the chromosomes that are found in other cells. Other cells contain forty-six chromosomes; the germ cells contain twenty-three.

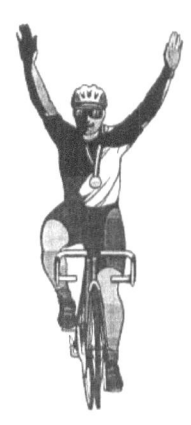

The reproductive organs can be divided into two main groups for both male and female: the gonads and accessory organs.

The gonads are sex glands that produce germ cells and hormones. The male gonads (testes) are located in the scrota, which are outside the male body, suspended between the thighs. The testes produce spermatozoa and secrete the male sex hormone, testosterone. Testosterone is deposited directly into the bloodstream, where it has three basic functions: to maintain the reproductive structures, to develop spermatozoa, and to develop secondary sex characteristics (traits that characterize males [e.g., deep voice, broad shoulders, narrow hips, more massive muscle tissues, and more body hair] as compared to those same traits in females). Spermatozoa are carried from the testes inside tubes called tubules. From the tubules, germ cells are collected and stored in the epididymis, where they mature and become able to move. The spermatozoa move through the ductus deferens, where they are carried to the duct of the seminal vesicle, where the ejaculatory duct enters the prostate glands. The spermatozoa are then emptied into the urethra.

Semen is a mixture of spermatozoa and secretions expelled by the prostate and Cowper's glands. Semen nourishes and transports spermatozoa, neutralizes acids in the female vaginal tract, and lubricates it by way of the penis. From this semen, at least two hundred million spermatozoa are released. Out of the millions, only one will live, if any, to reach the female ovum and fertilize. To allow intercourse, the penis is filled with blood, allowing it stiffen and enter the vagina.

The female gonads are called ovaries. This is where the female germ cells and hormones are produced. The ovaries protrude as far out as the pelvic portion of the female abdomen, where they are attached to the uterus and body wall. Female germ cells, ova, are discharged from the ovaries into two oviducts—egg-carrying tubes of the female reproductive system. The oviducts, also called fallopian tubes, move the ovum (a single ova) to the uterus. This process takes five days. The uterus is the area where a potential fetus grows to maturity and is released to the vagina. The vagina is the lower area of the birth canal that receives the penis during intercourse and where the mature fetus is contracted outside the female body.

The female reproductive system is cyclical (comes in cycles). Once each month, the ovum is released from the ovary, and the reproductive process resumes again. If a spermatozoon joins an ovum, fertilization takes place, and a fetus begins to develop.

The Body Systems

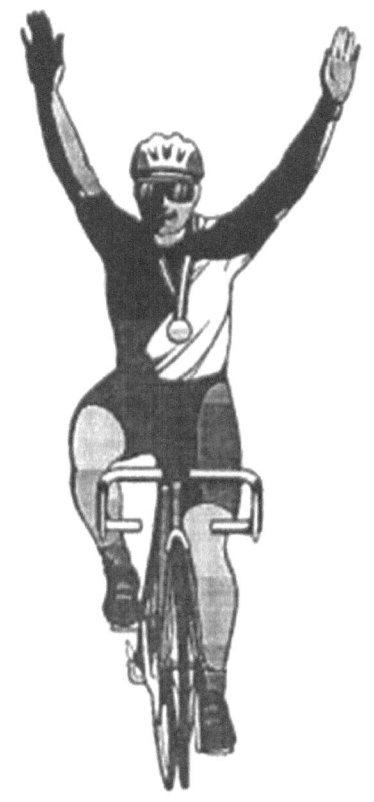

Worksheets

Worksheet 1

The Skeletal System

1. The frame of the body is called the _____ system.
2. The skeletal system consists of over _____ joints and bones.
3. _____ are the framework of the skeletal system.
4. Bones connect to other bones at points called _____.
5. Immovable joints are called _____ joints.
6. Slightly movable joints are called _____ joints.
7. _____ joints are freely movable.
8. The _____ skeleton consists of the skull, upper and lower jawbones, and neck bones.
9. The _____ includes the rib cage and pelvic, shoulder, and spinal bones.
10. The _____ limbs include the leg, foot, ankle, and toe bones and kneecaps.
11. The rib cage is located in the _____ trunk area.
12. The liver is located in the _____ trunk area.
13. The wrist bones are located in the _____ limbs.
14. The upper limbs allows for complicated _____.
15. The reproductive system is located in the _____ trunk area.

Worksheet 2

The Muscular System

1. A muscle is made up of _____.
2. Each muscle _____ is connected to a nerve.
3. Nerves receive instructions from the _____ and relay the information to the muscles.
4. There are _____ kinds of muscle tissues.
5. Muscles are either voluntary or _____.
6. _____ muscles control body movement.
7. _____ muscles such as the arteries are involuntary.
8. The _____ muscles are the strongest muscles in the body.
9. _____ muscles pump blood to the body's circulatory system.
10. Muscles that work against each other are called _____ muscles.
11. Involuntary muscles work without _____ commands from the brain.
12. Muscles _____ due to their ability to make themselves shorter and fatter.
13. When muscles become shorter and fatter, they perform a task called _____.
14. In antagonistic muscles, the moving muscle is called the _____ mover.
15. In antagonistic muscles, the relaxed muscle is called the _____.

Worksheet 3

The Digestive System

1. The _____ system allows for movement.
2. The _____ system consists basically of the alimentary canal.
3. The _____ system is the framework of our body.
4. One continuous tube that connects the mouth and all organs between it and the anal opening is called the _____.
5. _____ form organs.
6. A group of _____ working together form body systems.
7. Food is grounded and mixed with saliva to prepare it for digestion in the _____.
8. The _____ carries food from the mouth to the stomach.
9. The _____ is an organ that breaks down protein.
10. Hydrochloric acid is secreted to activate _____, an enzyme.
11. The absorption of water from the body's waste and by-products takes place in the _____.
12. The _____ secretes enzymes into the stomach to break down proteins, starches, and fats.
13. Undigested materials from the small intestine are passed to the _____.
14. Bile is secreted to the stomach by the _____.
15. Nutrients from digested foods pass through the small intestine and enter the body's _____.

Worksheet 4

The Circulatory System

1. The _____ system is a one-way transport system that carries blood throughout the body.
2. The _____ is the center of the circulatory system.
3. Hemoglobin is another word for _____.
4. Hemoglobin is composed of plasma, red blood cells, white blood cells, and _____.
5. The heart consists of _____ chambers.
6. The right _____ receives deoxygenated blood from the right atrium.
7. The right _____ pumps deoxygenated blood into the _____.
8. Oxygenated blood flows from the lungs to the left _____.
9. Oxygenated blood from the left atrium becomes deoxygenated in the left _____.
10. Hemoglobin is pumped from the heart into blood _____, which transfer the blood to other body organs.
11. There are _____ kinds of blood vessels.
12. The _____ are the smallest blood vessels.
13. _____ carry blood away from the heart.
14. Capillaries supply nutrient and oxygen to the body's _____.
15. The circulatory system also helps regulate the body's _____ by keeping it cool.

Worksheet 5

The Respiratory System

1. When nutrients are converted to energy, _____ respiration takes place.
2. he respiratory system consists of cartilage, tubes, and _____.
3. Cellular respiration has _____ phases.
4. The _____ is a muscle that carries air into the respiratory tract.
5. The _____ serves in the production of speech.
6. The _____ conducts air between the larynx and lungs.
7. The trachea divides into two branches called _____.
8. The _____ fills with air and passes oxygen to the capillaries.
9. The body has _____ lungs.
10. The sac that surrounds each lung is called the _____.
11. _____ takes place when air moves in and out of the lungs.
12. _____ takes place when oxygen is passed in the capillaries to the blood cells.
13. The expelling of carbon dioxide from the blood cells is also a process of _____.
14. When oxygen moves to the cells and carbon dioxide moves from the cells to the lungs, _____ takes place.
15. A dome-shaped muscle that serves as a partition between the lungs and abdominal cavity is called the _____.

Worksheet 6

The Nervous System

1. The _____ system is the main coordinating body system.
2. The _____ system receives messages from the other systems to be analyzed and transmits instruction back to these other systems.
3. The _____ system is composed of the brain, spinal cord, and nerves.
4. CNS refers to the _____ nervous system.
5. PNS refers to the _____ nervous system.
6. The brain and _____ form the central nervous system.
7. The _____ is located inside the cranial cavity.
8. Three layers of connective tissue that cover the brain are called _____.
9. About _____% of the body's oxygen is used by the brain.
10. Speech, smell, and memory are examples of actions that are regulated by the _____.
11. The brain _____ connects the brain and spinal cord.
12. The medulla _____ regulates breathing, heartbeat rate, blood flow, swallowing, and vomiting.
13. Nerves act as _____ devices that send messages.
14. _____ nerves conduct impulses to the brain.
15. _____ nerves conduct impulses away from the nerves.

Worksheet 7

The Integumentary System

1. Sweat and oil glands can be found in the _____ system.
2. The _____ system protects the other body systems.
3. The integumentary system is composed of _____, hair, nails, and sweat and oil glands.
4. The skin is an elastic-like _____ that covers the body.
5. The skin consists of _____ main layers.
6. The surface layer of the skin is called the _____.
7. _____ is a pigment that gives skin color.
8. The _____ is the second layer of tissue under the skin.
9. The _____ consists of connective tissue that contains muscles, nerves, capillaries, oil glands, and sweat glands.
10. A layer of tissue under the dermis is called the _____ layer.
11. _____ glands secrete sebum, which helps keep skin elastic.
12. Sweat glands are also called _____ glands.
13. Hair and nails are _____ of the integumentary system.
14. _____ are protective structures found on the fingers and toes.
15. The _____ from sweat glands, when modified by bacteria, produces body odor.

Worksheet 8

The Urinary System

1. The urinary system has _____ main organs.
2. The urinary system is sometimes referred to as the _____ system.
3. The body has _____ kidneys.
4. _____ act as filters.
5. _____ is liquid waste produced in and excreted by the kidneys.
6. The kidneys produce _____ that regulate blood pressure and prevent anemia.
7. A tube that carries urine from the kidneys to the bladder is called _____.
8. The _____ is a temporary reservoir for holding urine.
9. A tube extending from the bladder to the outside of the body is called a/an _____.
10. The body has _____ ureters that carry urine from the kidney to the bladder.
11. Ammonia, urea, uric acid, potassium, and sodium are all substances found in _____.
12. The _____ is a part of the male reproductive system.
13. In the female, the urethra serves _____ function.
14. The primary function of the _____ system is to excrete body waste and excessive water from the body.
15. The male _____ carries semen during ejaculation and urine on other occasions.

Worksheet 9

The Endocrine System

1. The _____ system produces hormones.
2. _____ are chemical messengers.
3. Hormones help _____ body functions.
4. Hormones are released into tissue fluid and the _____ stream.
5. Hormones are made of either protein or _____.
6. Most hormones are made of _____.
7. Adrenal cortex glands and sex glands are made up of _____ hormones.
8. The _____ glands produce thyroxine.
9. The _____ glands produce epinephrine and glucocorticoid.
10. The _____ glands secrete parathyroid hormone.
11. The pancreas secretes _____ and insulin.
12. Insulin is a _____ secreted by the pancreas.
13. _____ is the main male sex hormone.
14. _____ is a female hormone.
15. The _____ glands help stimulate other glands and secrete antidiuretic hormones.

Worksheet 10

The Reproductive System

1. The reproductive system is essential for the _____ of the human species.
2. Male sex cells are called _____.
3. The female sex cell is called a/an_____.
4. Sex cells contain _____ chromosomes.
5. All other human cells contain _____ chromosomes.
6. _____ are sex glands that produce germ cells and hormones.
7. _____ cells are sex cells.
8. The male gonads are called _____.
9. The female gonads are called _____.
10. It takes _____ days to move the ovum to the uterus.
11. The _____ is the lower area of the birth canal and receives the penis during intercourse.
12. For a woman, the reproductive cycle comes _____ each month.
13. _____ is a mixture of spermatozoa and secretions expelled by the prostate and Cowper's glands.
14. At least _____ million spermatozoa are released each time a male has intercourse.
15. The fetus grows to mature in the female _____.

Vocabulary Worksheet

Unit 1
The Skeletal System

Define the following terms in your own words:

1. Bones

_____

_____

_____

2. Joints

_____

_____

_____

3. Fibrous joints

_____

_____

_____

4. Cartilaginous joints

_____

_____

_____

5. Synovial joints

_____

_____

_____

6. Skeletal system

_____

_____

_____

7. Cranial skeleton

_____

_____

_____

8. Upper limbs

_____

_____

_____

9. Lower limbs

_____

_____

_____

10. Trunk

_____

_____

_____

Vocabulary Worksheet

Unit 2
The Muscular System

Define the following terms in your own words:

1. Muscles

_____

_____

_____

2. Skeletal muscles

_____

_____

_____

3. Voluntary muscles

_____

_____

_____

4. Smooth muscles

_____

_____

_____

5. Involuntary muscles

_____

_____

_____

6. Cardiac muscles

_____

_____

_____

Vocabulary Worksheet

Unit 3
The Digestive System

Define the following terms in your own words:

1. Digestive system

_____

_____

_____

2. Alimentary canal

_____

_____

_____

3. Bile

_____

_____

_____

4. Amylase

_____

_____

_____

5. Esophagus

_____

_____

_____

6. Stomach

_____

_____

_____

Vocabulary Worksheet

Unit 4
The Circulatory System

Define the following terms in your own words:

1. Circulatory system

_____

_____

_____

2. Hemoglobin

_____

_____

_____

3. Coagulation

_____

_____

_____

4. Right atrium

_____

_____

_____

5. Left atrium

_____

_____

_____

6. Right ventricle

_____

_____

_____

7. Left ventricle

_____

_____

_____

8. Capillaries

_____

_____

_____

9. Arteries

_____

_____

_____

10. Veins

_____

_____

_____

Vocabulary Worksheet

Unit 5
The Respiratory System

Define the following terms in your own words:

1. Respiratory system

_____

_____

_____

2. Ventilation

_____

_____

_____

3. Diffusion

_____

_____

_____

4. Transport

_____

_____

_____

5. Pharynx

_____

_____

_____

6. Larynx

_____

_____

_____

7. Trachea

_____

_____

_____

8. Bronchi

_____

_____

_____

9. Diaphragm

_____

_____

_____

10. Cellular respiration

_____

_____

_____

Vocabulary Worksheet

Unit 6
The Nervous System

Define the following terms in your own words:

1. Homeostasis

_____

_____

_____

2. Nervous system

_____

_____

_____

3. Brain

_____

_____

_____

4. Spinal cord

_____

_____

_____

5. Nerves

_____

_____

_____

6. Reflex actions

_____

_____

_____

7. Meninges

_____

_____

_____

8. Pons

_____

_____

_____

9. Medulla oblongata

_____

_____

_____

10. Afferent nerves

_____

_____

_____

Vocabulary Worksheet

Unit 7
The Integumentary System

Define the following terms in your own words:

1. Integumentary system

_____

_____

_____

2. Dermis

_____

_____

_____

3. Epidermis

_____

_____

_____

4. Membrane

_____

_____

_____

5. Melanin

_____

_____

_____

6. Subcutaneous layer

_____

_____

_____

7. Sebaceous glands

_____

_____

_____

8. Sudoriferous glands

_____

_____

_____

9. Keratin

_____

_____

_____

10. Sebum

_____

_____

_____

Vocabulary Worksheet

Unit 8
The Urinary System

Define the following terms in your own words:

1. Excretory system

_____

_____

_____

2. Kidneys

_____

_____

_____

3. Urine

_____

_____

_____

4. Ureters

_____

_____

_____

5. Peristalsis

_____

_____

_____

6. Urinary bladder

_____

_____

_____

7. Urethra

_____

_____

_____

8. Excrete

_____

_____

_____

9. Urea

_____

_____

_____

10. Anemia

_____

_____

_____

Vocabulary Worksheet

Unit 9
The Endocrine System

Define the following terms in your own words:

1. Endocrine system

_____

_____

_____

2. Hormones

_____

_____

_____

3. Thyroid glands

_____

_____

_____

4. Thyroxine

_____

_____

_____

5. Calcitonin

_____

_____

_____

6. Parathyroid glands

_____

_____

_____

7. Adrenal glands

_____

_____

_____

8. Pancreas

_____

_____

_____

9. Pituitary glands

_____

_____

_____

10. Testosterone

_____

_____

_____

Vocabulary Worksheet

Unit 10
The Reproductive System

Define the following terms in your own words:

1. Reproductive system

_____

_____

_____

2. Germ cells

_____

_____

_____

3. Spermatozoa

_____

_____

_____

4. Gonads

_____

_____

_____

5. Testes

_____

_____

_____

6. Ovaries

_____

_____

_____

7. Cowper's glands

_____

_____

_____

8. Ova

_____

_____

_____

9. Oviduct

_____

_____

_____

10. Fertilization

_____

_____

_____

Body Systems

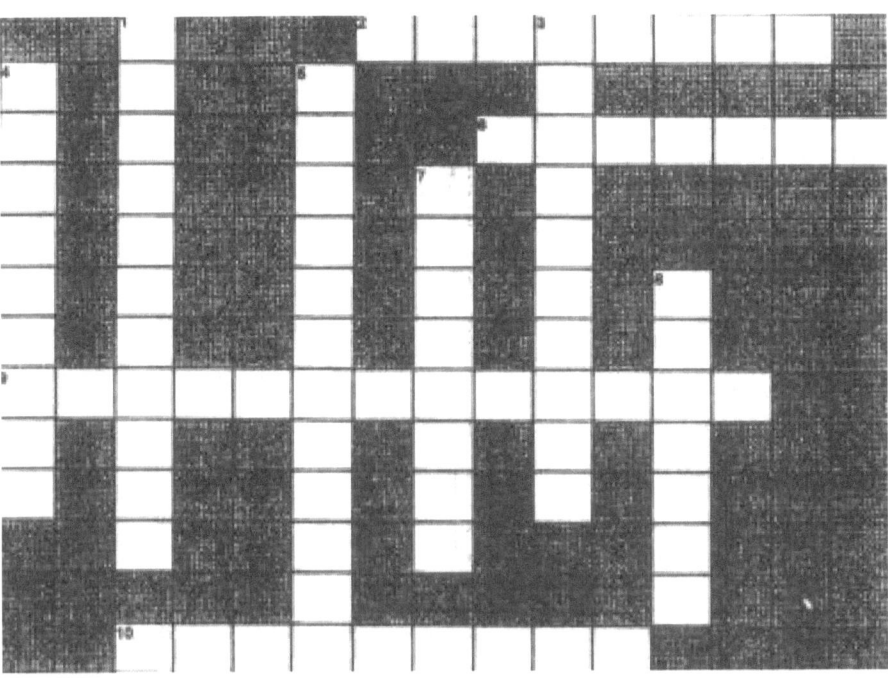

Across

2. Biceps

6. Ureter

9. Skin

10. Colon

Down

1. Lung

3. Heart

4. Glands

5. Embryo

7. Spine

8. Brain

Skeletal System

T	E	M	P	O	R	A	L	B	O	N	E	D	A	V
N	M	L	E	N	S	M	S	U	L	N	A	L	E	C
I	U	A	M	T	C	Y	U	M	M	A	U	R	I	B
O	N	C	O	U	A	R	S	T	Y	B	T	C	H	S
J	R	I	Y	I	P	C	R	O	I	E	A	A	S	U
C	E	V	W	Z	U	A	A	F	B	R	P	R	U	R
A	T	R	L	H	L	S	T	R	O	X	U	P	I	E
I	S	E	G	N	A	L	A	H	P	M	B	U	D	M
L	E	C	L	B	H	E	T	O	E	U	I	S	A	U
I	C	O	C	C	Y	X	E	F	R	D	S	N	R	H
O	V	T	Q	U	I	Z	M	V	T	N	D	U	K	X
R	W	C	M	L	I	V	A	L	L	I	X	A	M	Y
C	P	A	T	E	L	L	A	D	B	G	B	G	I	K
A	R	D	R	X	K	W	Z	L	N	B	U	I	N	R
S	Q	K	L	Q	H	Z	E	F	C	C	E	W	A	G

carpus	pubis	lumbar	temporal bone
cervical	radius	mandible	thoracic
clavicle	rib	maxilla	tibia
coccyx	sacroiliac joint	metacarpus	ulna
femur	sacrym	metatarsus	vertebrae
fibula	scapula	patella	
humerus	sternum	phalanges	

Muscular System

S	I	R	O	M	E	F	S	U	T	C	E	R	A	B
S	I	R	O	S	I	R	A	L	U	C	I	B	R	O
R	S	T	E	R	N	O	H	Y	O	I	D	E	I	Y
T	E	M	P	R	O	R	A	L	M	U	S	C	L	E
Z	J	Z	S	U	E	N	I	T	C	E	P	Z	P	T
V	A	S	T	U	S	L	A	T	E	R	A	L	I	S
Y	Z	G	A	S	T	R	O	C	N	E	M	I	U	S
S	U	I	R	O	T	R	A	S	P	E	C	I	R	T
G	R	A	C	I	L	I	S	D	E	L	T	O	I	D
P	E	C	T	O	R	A	L	I	S	M	A	J	O	R
F	R	O	N	T	A	L	M	U	S	C	L	E	G	L
Z	S	G	R	E	T	E	S	S	A	M	P	Q	H	U
S	U	I	Z	E	P	A	R	T	S	P	E	C	I	B
S	I	L	A	I	D	A	R	O	I	H	C	A	R	B
S	I	L	A	I	D	E	M	S	U	T	S	A	V	N

abductor longus   temproral muscle   masseter

biceps   trapezius   orbicularis oris

brachioradialis   triceps   pectineus

deltoid   vastus lateralis   pectoralis major

frontal muscle   vastus medialis   rectus femoris

gastrocnemius   sartorius

gracilis   sternohyoid

Word Search

Support, Movement, and Protection

Find the words from the list below in the puzzle and circle them.

(Contains backwards words.)

L	A	A	E	T	M	Q	N	X	O	R	N	O	I	A	B	A	R
A	E	D	S	T	F	H	R	F	C	L	L	F	O	M	N	O	A
R	D	T	I	E	A	T	Q	F	Q	D	E	C	I	A	I	W	C
Y	E	V	N	P	L	L	S	K	M	M	S	I	E	R	V	L	N
N	M	I	T	E	O	U	I	A	Z	A	R	O	E	K	V	N	E
X	A	B	H	G	P	S	C	D	F	O	M	T	K	Y	X	S	L
O	U	I	F	W	G	I	E	A	C	Y	N	I	K	J	N	D	B
F	K	F	L	A	M	R	T	S	M	A	C	V	B	J	V	L	I
J	B	S	J	B	B	G	U	H	C	J	Z	I	D	Z	U	W	R
X	W	C	L	M	D	O	C	A	E	A	A	W	M	P	P	Z	W
Y	I	L	Z	W	E	A	L	R	S	L	T	Y	T	N	U	F	L
F	Y	Y	M	S	R	C	V	Y	T	K	I	R	S	R	O	N	D
N	I	J	S	D	A	E	W	H	R	S	Y	A	O	P	G	P	M
W	W	O	I	N	P	U	X	V	D	K	S	Z	???	P	O	H	P
C	R	A	F	A	F	R	S	F	T	Y	N	I	I	E	H	I	X

Across

1. Inflammation of the urinary bladder

4. Inflammation of the liver

7. Accessory organ of the digestive tract that produces

Down

1. The outer layer of the kidney; contains most of the nephrons

2. Difficult or painful breathing

Name _____

Date _____

Career Planning—Puzzle 2

Find the listed words in the puzzle and circle them.

(Contains backwards words.)

O	Q	D	E	N	A	A	M	Z	L	F	M	U	D	Z	T	H	C	W	Z
K	N	M	O	F	Y	Y	T	I	C	V	S	R	B	Z	B	L	X	R	B
T	Q	C	M	M	X	T	C	T	R	Z	X	C	F	V	B	I	W	V	N
O	I	G	O	V	N	Y	I	C	E	E	U	K	N	E	X	R	E	F	I
E	D	F	A	U	Q	T	P	L	O	N	F	S	W	H	R	Z	R	E	M
R	X	W	M	P	T	T	A	Z	I	V	D	E	Y	H	V	X	B	Z	C
B	L	C	V	Z	W	Z	K	Z	N	B	E	A	R	G	M	K	F	A	Z
M	X	D	F	N	S	P	S	G	Y	C	A	R	N	E	H	H	C	Y	W
P	W	S	J	Q	Z	P	B	P	O	W	I	D	L	C	N	A	P	O	E
K	B	X	F	P	K	B	Z	O	E	N	I	G	N	E	E	C	X	Y	Y
G	F	Y	K	K	Q	N	P	C	I	N	J	E	R	E	T	R	E	V	O
U	Y	Z	F	N	U	E	N	T	T	B	D	S	E	Z	P	T	X	S	Q
D	W	S	Y	K	R	A	I	E	V	P	Z	G	H	Z	S	E	E	E	G
D	F	H	A	A	R	A	G	P	S	B	E	X	V	I	Y	V	D	R	T
S	L	M	T	A	T	R	E	Z	R	C	A	E	S	D	Y	M	L	Y	Z
T	P	I	E	I	I	Q	E	N	O	J	Y	B	M	L	Q	I	N	X	B
C	O	P	V	T	U	E	K	R	Q	O	G	D	D	D	W	R	W	D	O
N	P	E	Y	V	L	I	C	V	S	Y	L	M	P	K	Z	G	G	I	J
A	W	F	O	F	X	V	X	P	C	K	A	O	P	E	M	U	S	E	R
Y	S	X	U	T	W	N	U	R	L	I	V	D	R	R	E	E	R	A	C

APPEARANCE INITIATIVE

ATTENDANCE INTEGRITY

CAREER COOPERATION

JOB REFERENCES

COVER LETTER RESUME

DEPENDABILITY

Name _____

Date _____

Introduction to Medical Terminology—Puzzle 2

Find the listed words in the puzzle and circle them.

(Contains backwards words.)

K	C	W	Z	O	X	D	B	M	T	H	Y	N	V	G	O
X	D	D	M	A	H	R	O	H	P	W	M	Z	G	W	F
X	D	L	I	Y	E	R	R	D	Z	B	P	K	W	O	M
T	U	B	P	C	T	O	L	Z	D	M	B	V	B	M	V
P	A	E	S	S	M	H	R	T	X	M	B	T	A	A	N
L	R	I	A	B	C	J	E	X	V	P	C	N	Z	N	P
J	V	G	O	Z	T	I	P	P	M	W	S	F	D	T	J
Q	O	G	O	H	H	M	S	I	A	G	Z	I	K	O	A
M	B	X	Y	K	N	U	F	C	E	T	O	Y	R	C	D
J	V	R	X	J	E	T	G	T	I	G	J	G	F	W	R
T	N	A	P	Y	N	F	Y	H	X	R	N	U	I	V	L
Y	Y	Q	Z	E	E	K	Z	I	U	J	T	I	X	L	Q
U	R	I	A	M	H	L	Q	V	P	K	S	A	N	T	O
J	N	U	A	A	I	S	N	A	O	P	Y	H	I	E	A
R	S	R	V	Y	A	V	R	P	Y	S	O	T	C	E	M
S	O	M	A	T	L	L	I	T	Q	U	B	A	Q	K	Q

ECTO	MENING
GASTRO	OLIGO
HEPAT	PULMO
HYPER	SOMA
HYPO	THROMBO
IATRICS	URIA
JUXTA	USCER
IABIA	

Name _____

Date _____

Infection Control—Puzzle 2

Find the listed words in the puzzle and circle them.

(Contains backwards words.)

N	K	A	R	T	D	A	H	V	R	C	T	M	E	V	D	B	E
O	E	N	I	P	K	G	Q	K	N	Y	A	Q	I	I	A	W	Y
S	P	L	H	D	Q	C	R	B	D	A	T	R	U	C	Y	L	X
O	H	A	C	P	S	D	D	C	F	G	U	L	T	A	G	G	P
C	O	B	K	Y	A	M	S	W	W	S	F	E	X	F	F	E	A
O	O	V	S	L	C	T	E	W	M	C	R	J	D	T	F	S	Z
M	U	X	J	G	K	N	S	Y	I	I	N	L	F	H	R	N	S
I	R	T	F	R	U	P	O	T	A	N	T	A	G	X	J	E	I
A	C	R	W	E	E	X	O	I	C	S	T	Q	X	U	U	G	T
L	X	G	P	A	F	I	D	Y	T	I	R	M	X	O	K	O	I
I	O	L	W	U	N	S	E	J	U	C	B	E	H	D	V	H	T
D	T	A	H	M	I	A	J	H	F	W	E	O	I	M	N	T	A
Q	G	V	A	S	G	Z	C	L	L	W	S	F	R	R	K	A	P
Y	D	E	P	Y	Y	U	J	N	J	Q	A	J	N	E	R	P	E
P	A	E	K	X	Z	Q	D	F	C	I	G	G	T	I	A	A	H
E	S	J	B	X	H	G	N	O	I	T	A	L	O	S	I	N	C
A	I	M	M	U	N	E	S	Y	S	T	E	M	Y	W	T	U	A
U	R	F	V	G	D	I	U	L	F	L	A	I	V	O	N	Y	S

AIDS   INFECTION CYCLE
AMNIOTIC FLUID   ISOLATION
ANAEROBIC   NOSOCOMIAL
ASEPSIS   PATHOGENS
BACTERIA   STAPH
CARRIERS   SYNOVIAL FLUID
HEPATITIS
IMMUNE SYSTEM

Name _____

Date _____

The Safe Workplace—Puzzle 2

Find the listed words in the puzzle and circle them.

(Contains backwards words.)

V	H	U	A	Q	O	X	Z	L	A	C	I	V	R	E	C	C	P
C	H	E	M	I	C	A	L	D	I	T	S	D	F	R	P	V	P
N	K	H	O	T	T	B	F	G	M	Z	O	R	L	R	C	E	P
L	O	R	E	D	X	D	V	W	Q	Z	Y	U	F	O	T	R	F
N	Y	F	M	V	S	R	Q	C	N	A	P	E	N	V	H	T	J
C	O	T	G	V	C	S	O	R	W	M	E	T	H	N	O	E	D
D	O	I	E	C	F	N	Z	X	N	G	U	Q	G	U	R	B	R
N	X	J	T	F	C	F	B	Q	N	S	J	U	I	P	A	R	P
H	V	A	F	A	A	Z	Z	A	I	U	D	V	A	C	C	A	V
X	S	S	Z	O	R	S	R	O	B	E	E	H	C	T	I	E	S
S	D	J	U	F	S	E	N	S	A	N	M	I	L	X	C	D	L
G	K	Q	I	N	X	S	C	C	Z	E	V	L	K	G	Y	A	I
U	C	K	F	D	M	O	K	A	R	K	W	M	M	L	D	N	A
C	M	J	O	O	P	T	E	O	L	A	Z	D	N	H	E	V	R
E	V	M	T	P	G	M	F	P	X	C	B	G	O	O	M	G	E
V	S	I	J	L	H	M	V	R	K	F	S	M	Y	Z	R	E	D
Q	O	E	O	L	F	Q	A	A	Y	Z	P	I	U	P	C	L	I
N	Y	M	V	W	L	S	D	F	B	P	P	L	D	L	F	F	S

CERVICAL	MOTION
CHEMICAL	RANGE
CONTUSIONS	SAFETY
CPR	SIDERAILS
DISC	THORACIC
LACERATION	VERTEBRAE
LUMBAR	

Name _____

Date _____

Disasters: Preparedness, Hazards, and Prevention—Puzzle 2

Find the listed words in the puzzle and circle them.

(Contains backwards words.)

D	O	P	S	B	P	F	J	G	M	G	M	H	E	E	N
H	I	S	L	Y	Z	T	D	L	D	P	M	B	W	S	I
A	M	S	H	L	S	X	I	Y	R	A	E	P	F	G	O
Z	P	R	A	A	X	U	Y	O	Y	Z	R	P	H	D	O
A	X	R	X	S	A	D	X	A	E	E	E	Z	N	W	T
R	Y	K	C	O	T	S	O	I	U	V	X	K	S	O	G
D	L	S	R	I	A	E	B	H	G	S	O	T	X	A	U
S	Y	O	H	U	S	K	R	E	N	Q	I	I	S	W	R
K	R	L	F	F	H	F	R	K	S	Z	C	S	P	R	F
J	J	X	O	L	N	L	Y	R	W	T	E	H	E	R	X
M	P	F	I	F	R	U	W	G	T	S	O	F	V	P	K
S	W	F	H	Y	D	O	R	R	S	N	H	S	D	B	M
A	Y	Y	R	M	M	I	I	M	O	O	Z	S	V	F	N
O	W	Y	G	W	E	A	E	E	F	Y	L	Z	O	Q	T
A	X	Y	W	H	G	N	A	U	Y	Z	U	Z	Y	I	U
X	G	M	B	E	T	K	G	H	G	R	N	K	W	B	N

ASBESTOS   NIOSH

ASSESSMENT   OSHA

DISASTER   TOXIC

HAZARDS   TRIAGE

Name _____

Date _____

Understanding the Patient as a Person—Puzzle 2

Find the listed words in the puzzle and circle them.

(Contains backwards words.)

O	N	M	T	P	V	X	Z	U	J	W	O	T	V	P	X	T	L
S	K	F	I	X	P	X	G	E	F	Q	Y	G	U	L	N	S	I
A	T	W	G	N	L	S	G	O	O	T	W	B	E	E	Z	U	G
U	S	R	F	T	W	X	X	S	W	B	E	C	M	L	Y	X	K
N	R	O	E	Y	H	G	Z	D	A	R	I	P	R	H	S	P	Y
Q	U	U	V	S	A	B	X	O	T	P	O	S	N	H	X	C	T
X	X	Q	E	R	S	W	J	Y	S	L	P	N	Q	O	S	Q	U
P	V	X	A	C	E	Z	Z	O	E	W	U	V	F	E	F	S	I
V	F	W	X	X	N	N	H	V	P	W	B	V	I	K	Z	E	N
X	X	O	A	A	D	E	E	S	T	Q	M	G	L	Z	Y	G	O
L	O	H	M	M	D	D	C	A	E	S	Z	A	L	I	P	A	I
A	U	A	J	M	L	O	Q	S	I	E	G	G	Q	S	K	T	S
C	W	A	C	A	O	E	X	C	E	X	D	P	L	K	U	S	S
A	X	W	I	G	G	J	O	H	H	L	E	I	B	U	R	E	E
M	O	C	J	F	M	Y	N	A	C	E	O	R	C	E	G	F	R
F	O	Q	T	V	L	F	K	B	J	P	H	D	O	I	F	I	P
S	S	O	X	I	D	A	X	S	P	X	L	Y	A	N	U	L	E
M	V	P	D	E	J	L	A	N	O	I	T	O	M	E	A	S	D

ADOLESCENCE	LIFE STAGES
ANOREXIA	NERVOSA
DEPRESSION	PUBERTY
DEVELOPMENT	SOCIAL
EMOTIONAL	STRESS
HOSPICE	SUICIDE

Name _____

Date _____

Basic First Aid—Puzzle 2

Find the listed words in the puzzle and circle them.

(Contains backwards words.)

E	C	C	H	Y	M	O	S	I	S	O	Z	N	S	C	T	A	N	D	Z
E	P	I	S	T	A	X	I	S	P	T	C	F	G	W	L	E	R	F	T
F	Z	M	L	P	R	D	V	P	Y	T	S	U	R	H	T	W	A	J	S
H	A	T	K	E	Q	A	U	A	Z	A	P	E	Y	J	G	J	J	E	P
F	N	D	X	K	J	Z	O	E	D	Z	D	Y	I	T	Q	V	I	S	Q
S	R	L	N	V	E	X	I	O	F	E	Q	I	O	F	B	Z	I	N	A
K	Y	A	E	M	Y	C	K	Y	Q	L	R	C	D	G	U	S	O	B	C
K	A	N	C	T	E	J	D	D	Z	W	T	Y	U	R	O	I	R	A	T
P	T	E	C	T	O	D	Q	K	O	W	G	X	E	R	S	A	R	K	Z
D	Z	G	V	O	U	D	I	K	X	L	N	P	C	L	S	D	B	Y	B
C	H	H	C	U	P	R	I	C	E	M	U	E	U	I	I	O	B	D	W
F	E	V	Z	C	T	E	E	T	A	Y	N	V	O	A	K	E	S	L	Y
B	P	W	U	W	S	T	C	L	N	L	A	N	C	V	U	Y	M	H	V
G	H	S	X	Z	S	O	L	T	O	A	E	A	E	T	M	J	A	E	R
E	L	K	S	P	G	O	R	K	M	G	R	R	S	X	Z	J	G	G	O
K	R	G	C	N	C	I	R	J	T	R	R	F	T	J	P	S	H	H	M
K	S	A	A	L	Q	F	D	O	E	V	J	O	N	T	E	O	B	K	H
K	X	R	K	H	P	O	X	S	Q	B	H	Y	L	A	A	I	G	V	J
C	G	J	B	K	V	I	T	R	F	S	I	N	Q	L	J	G	L	I	V
K	A	N	A	I	C	Z	D	M	V	V	Y	V	A	B	C	Z	F	T	R

ABRASION	JAW THRUST
ANTIDOTE	LOG ROLL
AVULSION	MEDIC ALERT TAG
CARDIAC ARREST	NECROSIS
ECCHYMOSIS	SEIZURE
EPISTAXIS	SYNCOPE
FRACTURE	

Name _____

Date _____

Excretion—Puzzle 2

Find the listed words in the puzzle and circle them.

(Contains backwards words.)

D	M	L	V	F	D	Q	V	D	G	U	B	T	E	E	F
I	X	U	I	I	J	P	S	N	D	D	Y	N	S	I	T
A	Q	B	N	P	L	C	T	G	T	I	I	A	B	Y	O
L	P	S	R	U	A	L	Q	H	Y	P	L	R	V	I	Y
Y	J	V	Q	O	J	S	I	L	U	Y	I	A	L	P	I
S	B	Y	N	J	N	E	E	S	M	N	I	E	C	J	W
I	H	T	I	P	N	C	J	A	O	O	Z	T	S	T	S
S	W	F	E	A	I	Z	H	G	C	M	Z	X	B	G	I
M	Q	X	V	I	R	N	E	I	A	E	V	C	E	I	T
C	Q	I	Q	A	O	N	L	M	O	R	C	B	U	X	I
A	L	C	I	R	A	W	A	W	O	L	H	U	D	M	N
P	F	L	H	I	T	Z	C	V	W	C	E	T	M	V	I
Y	I	P	X	K	L	H	Z	W	N	R	W	S	E	M	H
C	E	O	Y	L	Q	L	J	D	J	R	F	U	N	R	R
N	N	H	E	M	A	T	U	R	I	A	Z	T	G	Q	U
A	E	N	D	O	S	C	O	P	Y	Z	Z	T	P	W	G

AMYLASE	HEMATURIA
ANOXIA	JEJUNUM
BRONCHIOLES	LIPASE
CECUM	NEPHRON
CILIA	RHINITIS
DIALYSIS	SUPINE
ENDOSCOPY	URETHRA
FIBRINOGEN	VILLA

Name _____

Date _____

Word Search

Excretion

Find the words from the list below in the puzzle and circle them.

(Contains backwards words.)

L	X	A	Q	A	C	S	Z	R	Q	W	A	H	A	A	K
Z	I	M	L	C	T	V	Z	J	Q	I	S	M	N	R	L
O	J	P	U	L	Z	U	S	Y	L	E	Y	O	V	B	F
L	S	J	A	C	I	T	I	I	L	L	X	W	M	U	J
Z	M	R	Y	S	E	V	C	O	A	I	C	L	R	Z	B
Y	O	C	W	P	E	C	I	S	A	V	V	E	F	P	R
H	W	R	L	A	O	H	E	N	D	T	M	Z	H	O	M
K	E	D	M	Y	C	C	O	U	Z	U	C	L	M	N	S
S	O	O	R	N	E	R	S	G	R	Y	I	C	L	O	I
A	I	F	O	N	H	H	N	O	M	E	C	K	A	U	S
S	Q	R	I	P	S	K	B	J	D	U	T	Y	E	Z	Y
V	B	P	E	K	K	Z	D	O	T	N	N	H	I	Z	L
U	U	N	D	N	R	P	V	B	E	R	E	U	R	C	A
S	T	R	Q	S	S	I	T	I	N	I	H	R	J	A	I
F	I	B	R	O	G	E	N	U	M	D	F	I	T	E	D
H	E	M	A	T	U	R	I	A	K	G	Q	V	V	W	J

AMYLASE	HEMATURIA
ANOXIA	JEJUNUM
BRONCHIOLES	LIPASE
CECUM	NEPHRON
CILIA	RHINITIS
DIALYSIS	SUPINE
ENDOSCOPY	URETHRA
FIBROGEN	VILLA

Unit Test 1   Score _____
The Skeletal System

                          Pass [_]   Retake [_]

Student name _____ Date _____

                          Correct   Incorrect
1. (a)(b)(c)(d)(e)   [_]   [_]
2. (a)(b)(c)(d)(e)   [_]   [_]
3. (a)(b)(c)(d)(e)   [_]   [_]
4. (a)(b)(c)(d)(e)   [_]   [_]
5. (a)(b)(c)(d)(e)   [_]   [_]
6. (a)(b)(c)(d)(e)   [_]   [_]
7. (a)(b)(c)(d)(e)   [_]   [_]
8. (a)(b)(c)(d)(e)   [_]   [_]
9. (a)(b)(c)(d)(e)   [_]   [_]
10. (a)(b)(c)(d)(e)   [_]   [_]
11. (a)(b)(c)(d)(e)   [_]   [_]
12. (a)(b)(c)(d)(e)   [_]   [_]
13. (a)(b)(c)(d)(e)   [_]   [_]
14. (a)(b)(c)(d)(e)   [_]   [_]
15. (a)(b)(c)(d)(e)   [_]   [_]
16. (a)(b)(c)(d)(e)   [_]   [_]
17. (a)(b)(c)(d)(e)   [_]   [_]
18. (a)(b)(c)(d)(e)   [_]   [_]
19. (a)(b)(c)(d)(e)   [_]   [_]
20. (a)(b)(c)(d)(e)   [_]   [_]

Unit Test 2   Score _____

The Muscular System

                        Pass [ ]   Retake [ ]

Student name _____ Date _____

                        Correct   Incorrect

1. (a)(b)(c)(d)(e)   [ ]   [ ]

2. (a)(b)(c)(d)(e)   [ ]   [ ]

3. (a)(b)(c)(d)(e)   [ ]   [ ]

4. (a)(b)(c)(d)(e)   [ ]   [ ]

5. (a)(b)(c)(d)(e)   [ ]   [ ]

6. (a)(b)(c)(d)(e)   [ ]   [ ]

7. (a)(b)(c)(d)(e)   [ ]   [ ]

8. (a)(b)(c)(d)(e)   [ ]   [ ]

9. (a)(b)(c)(d)(e)   [ ]   [ ]

10. (a)(b)(c)(d)(e)   [ ]   [ ]

11. (a)(b)(c)(d)(e)   [ ]   [ ]

12. (a)(b)(c)(d)(e)   [ ]   [ ]

13. (a)(b)(c)(d)(e)   [ ]   [ ]

14. (a)(b)(c)(d)(e)   [ ]   [ ]

15. (a)(b)(c)(d)(e)   [ ]   [ ]

16. (a)(b)(c)(d)(e)   [ ]   [ ]

17. (a)(b)(c)(d)(e)   [ ]   [ ]

18. (a)(b)(c)(d)(e)   [ ]   [ ]

19. (a)(b)(c)(d)(e)   [ ]   [ ]

20. (a)(b)(c)(d)(e)   [ ]   [ ]

Unit Test 3   Score _____
The Digestive System

Pass [_]   Retake [_]

Student name _____ Date _____

	Correct	Incorrect
1. (a)(b)(c)(d)(e)	[_]	[_]
2. (a)(b)(c)(d)(e)	[_]	[_]
3. (a)(b)(c)(d)(e)	[_]	[_]
4. (a)(b)(c)(d)(e)	[_]	[_]
5. (a)(b)(c)(d)(e)	[_]	[_]
6. (a)(b)(c)(d)(e)	[_]	[_]
7. (a)(b)(c)(d)(e)	[_]	[_]
8. (a)(b)(c)(d)(e)	[_]	[_]
9. (a)(b)(c)(d)(e)	[_]	[_]
10. (a)(b)(c)(d)(e)	[_]	[_]
11. (a)(b)(c)(d)(e)	[_]	[_]
12. (a)(b)(c)(d)(e)	[_]	[_]
13. (a)(b)(c)(d)(e)	[_]	[_]
14. (a)(b)(c)(d)(e)	[_]	[_]
15. (a)(b)(c)(d)(e)	[_]	[_]
16. (a)(b)(c)(d)(e)	[_]	[_]
17. (a)(b)(c)(d)(e)	[_]	[_]
18. (a)(b)(c)(d)(e)	[_]	[_]
19. (a)(b)(c)(d)(e)	[_]	[_]
20. (a)(b)(c)(d)(e)	[_]	[_]

Unit Test 4   Score _____

The Circulatory System

Pass [_]   Retake [_]

Student name _____ Date _____

	Correct	Incorrect
1. (a)(b)(c)(d)(e)	[_]	[_]
2. (a)(b)(c)(d)(e)	[_]	[_]
3. (a)(b)(c)(d)(e)	[_]	[_]
4. (a)(b)(c)(d)(e)	[_]	[_]
5. (a)(b)(c)(d)(e)	[_]	[_]
6. (a)(b)(c)(d)(e)	[_]	[_]
7. (a)(b)(c)(d)(e)	[_]	[_]
8. (a)(b)(c)(d)(e)	[_]	[_]
9. (a)(b)(c)(d)(e)	[_]	[_]
10. (a)(b)(c)(d)(e)	[_]	[_]
11. (a)(b)(c)(d)(e)	[_]	[_]
12. (a)(b)(c)(d)(e)	[_]	[_]
13. (a)(b)(c)(d)(e)	[_]	[_]
14. (a)(b)(c)(d)(e)	[_]	[_]
15. (a)(b)(c)(d)(e)	[_]	[_]
16. (a)(b)(c)(d)(e)	[_]	[_]
17. (a)(b)(c)(d)(e)	[_]	[_]
18. (a)(b)(c)(d)(e)	[_]	[_]
19. (a)(b)(c)(d)(e)	[_]	[_]
20. (a)(b)(c)(d)(e)	[_]	[_]

Unit Test 5   Score _____
The Respiratory System

                    Pass [_]   Retake [_]

Student name _____ Date _____

                         Correct   Incorrect
1. (a)(b)(c)(d)(e)   [_]   [_]
2. (a)(b)(c)(d)(e)   [_]   [_]
3. (a)(b)(c)(d)(e)   [_]   [_]
4. (a)(b)(c)(d)(e)   [_]   [_]
5. (a)(b)(c)(d)(e)   [_]   [_]
6. (a)(b)(c)(d)(e)   [_]   [_]
7. (a)(b)(c)(d)(e)   [_]   [_]
8. (a)(b)(c)(d)(e)   [_]   [_]
9. (a)(b)(c)(d)(e)   [_]   [_]
10. (a)(b)(c)(d)(e)   [_]   [_]
11. (a)(b)(c)(d)(e)   [_]   [_]
12. (a)(b)(c)(d)(e)   [_]   [_]
13. (a)(b)(c)(d)(e)   [_]   [_]
14. (a)(b)(c)(d)(e)   [_]   [_]
15. (a)(b)(c)(d)(e)   [_]   [_]
16. (a)(b)(c)(d)(e)   [_]   [_]
17. (a)(b)(c)(d)(e)   [_]   [_]
18. (a)(b)(c)(d)(e)   [_]   [_]
19. (a)(b)(c)(d)(e)   [_]   [_]
20. (a)(b)(c)(d)(e)   [_]   [_]

Unit Test 6   Score _____
The Nervous System

                        Pass [_]   Retake [_]

Student name _____ Date _____

                        Correct   Incorrect

1. (a)(b)(c)(d)(e)   [_]   [_]

2. (a)(b)(c)(d)(e)   [_]   [_]

3. (a)(b)(c)(d)(e)   [_]   [_]

4. (a)(b)(c)(d)(e)   [_]   [_]

5. (a)(b)(c)(d)(e)   [_]   [_]

6. (a)(b)(c)(d)(e)   [_]   [_]

7. (a)(b)(c)(d)(e)   [_]   [_]

8. (a)(b)(c)(d)(e)   [_]   [_]

9. (a)(b)(c)(d)(e)   [_]   [_]

10. (a)(b)(c)(d)(e)   [_]   [_]

11. (a)(b)(c)(d)(e)   [_]   [_]

12. (a)(b)(c)(d)(e)   [_]   [_]

13. (a)(b)(c)(d)(e)   [_]   [_]

14. (a)(b)(c)(d)(e)   [_]   [_]

15. (a)(b)(c)(d)(e)   [_]   [_]

16. (a)(b)(c)(d)(e)   [_]   [_]

17. (a)(b)(c)(d)(e)   [_]   [_]

18. (a)(b)(c)(d)(e)   [_]   [_]

19. (a)(b)(c)(d)(e)   [_]   [_]

20. (a)(b)(c)(d)(e)   [_]   [_]

Unit Test 7   Score _____

The Integumentary System

Pass [_]   Retake [_]

Student name _____ Date _____

	Correct	Incorrect
1. (a)(b)(c)(d)(e)	[_]	[_]
2. (a)(b)(c)(d)(e)	[_]	[_]
3. (a)(b)(c)(d)(e)	[_]	[_]
4. (a)(b)(c)(d)(e)	[_]	[_]
5. (a)(b)(c)(d)(e)	[_]	[_]
6. (a)(b)(c)(d)(e)	[_]	[_]
7. (a)(b)(c)(d)(e)	[_]	[_]
8. (a)(b)(c)(d)(e)	[_]	[_]
9. (a)(b)(c)(d)(e)	[_]	[_]
10. (a)(b)(c)(d)(e)	[_]	[_]
11. (a)(b)(c)(d)(e)	[_]	[_]
12. (a)(b)(c)(d)(e)	[_]	[_]
13. (a)(b)(c)(d)(e)	[_]	[_]
14. (a)(b)(c)(d)(e)	[_]	[_]
15. (a)(b)(c)(d)(e)	[_]	[_]
16. (a)(b)(c)(d)(e)	[_]	[_]
17. (a)(b)(c)(d)(e)	[_]	[_]
18. (a)(b)(c)(d)(e)	[_]	[_]
19. (a)(b)(c)(d)(e)	[_]	[_]
20. (a)(b)(c)(d)(e)	[_]	[_]

Unit Test 8   Score _____

The Urinary System

                        Pass [_]   Retake [_]

Student name _____ Date _____

                        Correct   Incorrect

1. (a)(b)(c)(d)(e)   [_]   [_]

2. (a)(b)(c)(d)(e)   [_]   [_]

3. (a)(b)(c)(d)(e)   [_]   [_]

4. (a)(b)(c)(d)(e)   [_]   [_]

5. (a)(b)(c)(d)(e)   [_]   [_]

6. (a)(b)(c)(d)(e)   [_]   [_]

7. (a)(b)(c)(d)(e)   [_]   [_]

8. (a)(b)(c)(d)(e)   [_]   [_]

9. (a)(b)(c)(d)(e)   [_]   [_]

10. (a)(b)(c)(d)(e)   [_]   [_]

11. (a)(b)(c)(d)(e)   [_]   [_]

12. (a)(b)(c)(d)(e)   [_]   [_]

13. (a)(b)(c)(d)(e)   [_]   [_]

14. (a)(b)(c)(d)(e)   [_]   [_]

15. (a)(b)(c)(d)(e)   [_]   [_]

16. (a)(b)(c)(d)(e)   [_]   [_]

17. (a)(b)(c)(d)(e)   [_]   [_]

18. (a)(b)(c)(d)(e)   [_]   [_]

19. (a)(b)(c)(d)(e)   [_]   [_]

20. (a)(b)(c)(d)(e)   [_]   [_]

Unit Test 9   Score _____
The Endocrine System

                              Pass [_]   Retake [_]

Student name _____ Date _____

	Correct	Incorrect
1. (a)(b)(c)(d)(e)	[_]	[_]
2. (a)(b)(c)(d)(e)	[_]	[_]
3. (a)(b)(c)(d)(e)	[_]	[_]
4. (a)(b)(c)(d)(e)	[_]	[_]
5. (a)(b)(c)(d)(e)	[_]	[_]
6. (a)(b)(c)(d)(e)	[_]	[_]
7. (a)(b)(c)(d)(e)	[_]	[_]
8. (a)(b)(c)(d)(e)	[_]	[_]
9. (a)(b)(c)(d)(e)	[_]	[_]
10. (a)(b)(c)(d)(e)	[_]	[_]
11. (a)(b)(c)(d)(e)	[_]	[_]
12. (a)(b)(c)(d)(e)	[_]	[_]
13. (a)(b)(c)(d)(e)	[_]	[_]
14. (a)(b)(c)(d)(e)	[_]	[_]
15. (a)(b)(c)(d)(e)	[_]	[_]
16. (a)(b)(c)(d)(e)	[_]	[_]
17. (a)(b)(c)(d)(e)	[_]	[_]
18. (a)(b)(c)(d)(e)	[_]	[_]
19. (a)(b)(c)(d)(e)	[_]	[_]
20. (a)(b)(c)(d)(e)	[_]	[_]

Unit Test 10 Score _____
The Reproductive System

Pass [ ] Retake [ ]

Student name _____ Date _____

	Correct	Incorrect
1. (a)(b)(c)(d)(e)	[ ]	[ ]
2. (a)(b)(c)(d)(e)	[ ]	[ ]
3. (a)(b)(c)(d)(e)	[ ]	[ ]
4. (a)(b)(c)(d)(e)	[ ]	[ ]
5. (a)(b)(c)(d)(e)	[ ]	[ ]
6. (a)(b)(c)(d)(e)	[ ]	[ ]
7. (a)(b)(c)(d)(e)	[ ]	[ ]
8. (a)(b)(c)(d)(e)	[ ]	[ ]
9. (a)(b)(c)(d)(e)	[ ]	[ ]
10. (a)(b)(c)(d)(e)	[ ]	[ ]
11. (a)(b)(c)(d)(e)	[ ]	[ ]
12. (a)(b)(c)(d)(e)	[ ]	[ ]
13. (a)(b)(c)(d)(e)	[ ]	[ ]
14. (a)(b)(c)(d)(e)	[ ]	[ ]
15. (a)(b)(c)(d)(e)	[ ]	[ ]
16. (a)(b)(c)(d)(e)	[ ]	[ ]
17. (a)(b)(c)(d)(e)	[ ]	[ ]
18. (a)(b)(c)(d)(e)	[ ]	[ ]
19. (a)(b)(c)(d)(e)	[ ]	[ ]
20. (a)(b)(c)(d)(e)	[ ]	[ ]

Grade Sheet for Phase 1   The Body System

Student Name	Quiz 1	Quiz 2	Quiz 3	Quiz 4	Quiz 5	Quiz 6	Quiz 7	Quiz 8	Quiz 9	Quiz 10	Final Quiz	Aver.

The Skeletal System

Unit Test 1

1. The skeletal system can be compared to a _____.

    a. car
    b. movie
    c. horse
    d. telephone
    e. none of the above

2. The basic framework of the body is called the _____.

    a. cardiac system
    b. endocrine system
    c. skeletal system
    d. muscular system
    e. none of the above

3. Bones are composed of _____.

    a. tissues
    b. blood vessels
    c. nerves
    d. all of the above
    e. none of the above

4. Bones are connected by _____.

    a. ligaments
    b. nerves
    c. muscles
    d. joints
    e. none of the above

5. Bones are connected at the _____.

   a. ligaments
   b. nerves
   c. muscles
   d. joints
   e. none of the above

6. Immovable joints are _____.

   a. fibrous
   b. cartilaginous
   c. synovial
   d. skeletal
   e. none of the above

7. Freely movable joints are _____.

   a. fibrous
   b. cartilaginous
   c. synovial
   d. skeletal
   e. none of the above

8. The number of basic functions the skeletal system serves is _____.

   a. 5
   b. 8
   c. 7
   d. 2
   e. none of the above

9. The part of the skeleton that protects the liver, kidney, reproductive system, stomach, and pancreas is the _____.

    a. upper limbs
    b. lower limbs
    c. upper trunk
    d. lower trunk
    e. none of the above

10. Joints that are slightly movable are _____.

    a. cartilaginous
    b. cranial
    c. synovial
    d. both *a* and *c*
    e. none of the above

11. The weight of the cranial skeleton, trunk, and upper limbs is supported by the _____.

    a. spinal cord
    b. skull
    c. pelvic bone
    d. lower limbs
    e. none of the above

12. Functions of the bones include _____.

    a. the production of blood cells
    b. facilitation of skeletal movement
    c. storing of calcium
    d. all of the above
    e. none of the above

13. Wrist bones are part of the _____.

    a. cranial skeleton

    b. upper trunk

    c. lower trunk

    d. upper limbs

    e. none of the above

14. Touch is facilitated by the _____.

    a. cranial skeleton

    b. upper trunk

    c. lower trunk

    d. upper limbs

    e. none of the above

15. The arms are connected to the upper body by the _____.

    a. spinal cord

    b. lower limbs

    c. cranial skeleton

    d. lower trunk

    e. none of the above

16. All of the following except _____ are joint systems.

    a. mastoid joints

    b. fibrous joints

    c. cartilaginous joints

    d. synovial joints

    e. none of the above

The Muscular System

Unit Test 2

1. Muscles can be seen as the body's _____.

   a. framework
   b. movers
   c. workers
   d. digestive system
   e. none of the above

2. There are more than _____ individual muscles in the human body.

   a. 650
   b. 60
   c. 1000
   d. 25
   e. none of the above

3. Muscles work in _____ by pulling.

   a. sections
   b. place
   c. composition
   d. pairs
   e. none of the above

4. Muscles compose nearly _____ of our body weight.

   a. 95%
   b. 90%
   c. 9%
   d. 25%
   e. none of the above

5. The body has _____ kinds of muscle tissues.

    a. 2
    b. 4
    c. 6
    d. 8
    e. none of the above

6. Skeletal muscles are _____ muscles (controlled by will).

    a. involuntary
    b. reflex
    c. smooth muscles
    d. not controlled by will
    e. none of the above

7. The skeletal muscle tissue controls body _____.

    a. movement
    b. temperature
    c. circulation
    d. consciousness
    e. none of the above

8. Smooth muscles are _____ muscles.

    a. involuntary
    b. voluntary
    c. the strongest
    d. all of the above
    e. none of the above

9. Arteries are examples of a _____ muscle tissue.

    a. skeletal
    b. smooth
    c. cardiac
    d. all of the above
    e. none of the above

10. The _____ muscle is the strongest muscle in the body.

    a. skeletal
    b. smooth
    c. cardiac
    d. artery
    e. none of the above

11. The cardiac muscle tissue is _____.

    a. skeletal
    b. smooth
    c. involuntary
    d. all of the above
    e. none of the above

12. Cardiac muscles pump blood to the body's _____ system.

    a. skeletal
    b. heart
    c. muscle
    d. circulatory
    e. none of the above

13. All muscles _____.

    a. bend

    b. pull

    c. pump blood

    d. move bones

    e. none of the above

14. The muscles pull because of their ability to make themselves _____ and fatter.

    a. shorter

    b. larger

    c. stronger

    d. all of the above

    e. none of the above

15. Every bone or organ in the body that moves, pumps, or pushes is controlled by a _____ of muscles.

    a. skeletal

    b. voluntary

    c. smooth

    d. pair of

    e. none of the above

16. Involuntary muscles are not controlled by _____.

    a. blood

    b. organs

    c. will

    d. tissue

    e. none of the above

17. Cardiac muscles work without _____ commands from the mind.

   a. conscious
   b. involuntary
   c. skeletal
   d. unconscious
   e. none of the above

18. When muscles pull, this is called _____.

   a. contraction
   b. pulling
   c. circulation
   d. will power
   e. none of the above

19. Muscles allow _____ or organs to move, pump, or push.

   a. cardiac tissue
   b. skeletal tissue
   c. smooth tissue
   d. bones
   e. none of the above

20. Both cardiac and smooth muscles are _____.

   a. related
   b. controlled
   c. involuntary
   d. voluntary
   e. none of the above

The Digestive System

Unit Test 3

1. The digestive system consists basically of the _____.

   a. anal
   b. alimentary canal
   c. liver
   d. mouth
   e. none of the above

2. The alimentary canal connects the mouth and all organs between it to the _____ opening.

   a. anal
   b. liver
   c. pancreas
   d. intestine
   e. none of the above

3. Cells form _____.

   a. acids
   b. protein
   c. pepsin
   d. organs
   e. none of the above

4. A group of organs working together to perform a specific function form _____ systems.

   a. digestive
   b. cell
   c. tissue
   d. organ
   e. none of the above

5. The digestive system is an _____ system.

   a. selective
   b. cellular
   c. tissue
   d. organ
   e. none of the above

6. The digestive system is composed of _____ basic organs.

   a. 7
   b. 8
   c. 9
   d. 6
   e. none of the above

7. The _____ is used to prepare food for digestion.

   a. esophagus
   b. mouth
   c. liver
   d. anal canal
   e. none of the above

8. _____ is a component of saliva that lubricates foods.

   a. Hydrochloric acid
   b. Mucus
   c. Pepsin
   d. Enzymes
   e. None of the above

9. The _____ is a tubelike organ that carries food from the mouth to the stomach.

   a. esophagus
   b. liver
   c. pancreas
   d. intestine
   e. none of the above

10. The _____ is the organ in the digestive system that breaks down protein.

   a. protein
   b. liver
   c. stomach
   d. esophagus
   e. none of the above

11. Pepsin is an _____ that helps break down protein.

   a. protein
   b. mucus
   c. hormone
   d. enzyme
   e. none of the above

12. The stomach secretes _____ to neutralize acids.

    a. acid

    b. minerals

    c. mucus

    d. bacteria

    e. none of the above

13. The small _____ absorbs the water from the by-product of the stomach.

    a. pancreas

    b. intestine

    c. esophagus

    d. liver

    e. none of the above

14. Undigested materials pass through the large _____ and out of the anal opening.

    a. liver

    b. pancreas

    c. stomach

    d. esophagus

    e. none of the above

15. The _____ is a body organ that secretes enzymes in to the stomach.

    a. pancreas

    b. liver

    c. esophagus

    d. intestine

    e. none of the above

16. The _____ is a body organ that secretes bile from the gall bladder into the stomach.

   a. bladder

   b. pancreas

   c. esophagus

   d. liver

   e. none of the above

17. _____ breaks up large fat globules into smaller droplets.

   a. Hydrochloric acid

   b. Mucus

   c. Pepsin

   d. Bile

   e. None of the above

18. Once food has been digested, nutrients pass through the small intestine and into the _____.

   a. liver

   b. large intestine

   c. bloodstream

   d. stomach

   e. none of the above

19. All except for the _____ are organs of the digestive system.

   a. liver

   b. kidney

   c. heart

   d. pancreas

   e. none of the above

20. Saliva contains about _____ water.

    a. 50%
    b. 75%
    c. 85%
    d. 90%
    e. none of the above

The Circulatory System

Unit Test 4

1. The circulatory system does all except _____.

   a. send nutrients to the body's cells
   b. conduct air between the larynx and the lungs
   c. send oxygen to the body's cells
   d. carry away cells' by-products
   e. none of the above

2. The circulatory system is a one-way transport system that carries _____throughout the body.

   a. blood
   b. hemoglobin
   c. thrombocyte
   d. all of the above
   e. none of the above

3. The center of the circulatory system is _____.

   a. the arteries
   b. the capillary
   c. the vein
   d. all of the above
   e. none of the above

4. The _____ is a muscle that consists of four chambers.

   a. artery

   b. capillary

   c. lung

   d. heart

   e. none of the above

5. Hemoglobin is also called _____.

   a. blood

   b. plasma

   c. white blood cells

   d. red blood cells

   e. none of the above

6. Hemoglobin is composed of _____.

   a. plasma

   b. white blood cells

   c. red blood cells

   d. all of the above

   e. none of the above

7. Cells that help blood coagulate are called _____.

   a. thrombocytes

   b. white blood cells

   c. red blood cells

   d. all of the above

   e. none of the above

8. The liquid portion of blood is called _____.

   a. hemoglobin
   b. thrombocyte
   c. plasma
   d. all of the above
   e. none of the above

9. The heart pumps blood into _____.

   a. capillaries
   b. veins
   c. arteries
   d. lungs
   e. none of the above

10. The left atrium receives _____ blood from the lungs.

   a. infectious
   b. deoxygenated
   c. thrombotic
   d. oxygenated
   e. none of the above

11. The right ventricle pumps _____ blood into the lung.

   a. infectious
   b. deoxygenated
   c. thrombotic
   d. oxygenated
   e. none of the above

12. Oxygenated blood is pumped into the _____.

    a. left ventricle

    b. right ventricle

    c. right atrium

    d. all of the above

    e. none of the above

13. Which of the items below is a blood vessel?

    a. arteries

    b. veins

    c. capillaries

    d. all of the above

    e. none of the above

14. _____ are blood vessels that carry blood away from the heart.

    a. Arteries

    b. Veins

    c. Capillaries

    d. All of the above

    e. None of the above

15. The smallest blood vessels are called _____.

    a. arteries

    b. veins

    c. capillaries

    d. valves

    e. none of the above

16. The blood vessel that transports carbon dioxide to the lungs is called
    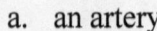.

   a. an artery
   b. a vein
   c. a capillary
   d. a valve
   e. none of the above

The Respiratory System

Unit Test 5

1. The respiratory system is composed of _____.

    a. cartilage
    b. tubes
    c. muscles
    d. all of the above
    e. none of the above

2. The respiratory system forms a _____ for air to be brought to cells and their by-products released in the atmosphere.

    a. chamber
    b. pathway
    c. branch
    d. cavity
    e. none of the above

3. Your body's nutrients are converted to _____.

    a. energy
    b. cells
    c. cartilage
    d. food
    e. none of the above

4. Cellular respiration has _____ phases.

   a. 4
   b. 6
   c. 3
   d. 9
   e. none of the above

5. One phase of cellular respiration is called _____.

   a. ventilation
   b. cellulization
   c. respiration
   d. all of the above
   e. none of the above

6. A muscle that carries air into the respiratory tract is called _____.

   a. larynx
   b. bronchus
   c. trachea
   d. pharynx
   e. none of the above

7. The _____ is a tube consisting of cartilage and chambers, which receives air from the pharynx.

   a. larynx
   b. bronchus
   c. trachea
   d. pharynx
   e. none of the above

8. Another word for windpipe is _____.

    a. thoracic
    b. larynx
    c. pharynx
    d. trachea
    e. none of the above

9. The _____ conducts air between the larynx and the lungs.

    a. thoracic
    b. larynx
    c. pharynx
    d. trachea
    e. none of the above

10. The right bronchus is _____ than the left bronchus.

    a. smaller
    b. lighter
    c. larger
    d. darker
    e. none of the above

11. The two bronchi enter the _____ and transport the air from the trachea to the lungs.

    a. lungs
    b. pharynx
    c. larynx
    d. vocal cords
    e. none of the above

12. The _____ serves in the production of speech.

    a. pharynx

    b. larynx

    c. trachea

    d. all of the above

    e. none of the above

13. All are phases of cellular respiration except _____.

    a. ventilation

    b. carbon dioxide

    c. diffusion

    d. transport

    e. none of the above

14. The blood vessels and _____ are also connected with each lung in its bronchus.

    a. lungs

    b. nerves

    c. cavies

    d. bronchi

    e. none of the above

15. Carbon dioxide is _____.

    a. water vapor

    b. gas

    c. cells

    d. a form of oxygen

    e. none of the above

16. A dome-shaped muscle that forms a partition between the lungs and the abdominal cavity is the _____.

    a. pleura
    b. trachea
    c. diaphragm
    d. alveoli
    e. none of the above

17. Each lung is covered by a closed sac called the _____.

    a. pleura
    b. diaphragm
    c. thoracic
    d. larynx
    e. none of the above

18. The movement of air in and out of the lungs is known as _____.

    a. transport
    b. diffusion
    c. conversion
    d. ventilation
    e. none of the above

19. When oxygen is passed in the capillaries to the blood cells and carbon dioxide is passed out of the blood cells, _____ takes place.

    a. transport
    b. diffusion
    c. conversion
    d. ventilation
    e. none of the above

20. When oxygen is moved to the cells and carbon dioxide moves from the cells to the lungs, this is called _____.

    a. transport
    b. diffusion
    c. ventilation
    d. all of the above
    e. none of the above

The Nervous System

Unit Test 6

1. All the body systems work _____ as one complete unit.

    a. interdependently
    b. independently
    c. consciously
    d. all of the above
    e. none of the above

2. The _____ system is the main coordinating system for the body.

    a. peripheral nervous
    b. nervous
    c. reflexive
    d. central nervous
    e. none of the above

3. The brain is covered by _____, fluids, and bones.

    a. membranes
    b. cartilage
    c. blood
    d. hormones
    e. none of the above

4. Messages that require quick responses are handled directly by the _____.

    a. peripheral nerves
    b. spinal cord
    c. brain stem
    d. midbrain
    e. none of the above

5. The _____ connects the midbrain to the medulla.

   a. medulla oblongata
   b. spinal cord
   c. peripheral nerves
   d. pons
   e. none of the above

6. The _____ nervous system is made up of nerves that control the actions of the skeletal muscles.

   a. central
   b. peripheral
   c. afferent
   d. somatic
   e. none of the above

The Integumentary System

Unit Test 7

1. The body is a complex system of _____.

   a. organs
   b. tissues
   c. nerves
   d. all of the above
   e. none of the above

2. The integumentary system is the body system designed to protect _____.

   a. other organs
   b. other body systems
   c. the nervous system
   d. all of the above
   e. none of the above

3. The skin is an elastic-like _____ that covers the body.

   a. dermis
   b. melanin
   c. epidermis
   d. all of the above
   e. none of the above

4. The skin consists of two main layers, the _____.

   a. sweat glands and oil gland
   b. epidermis and dermis
   c. keratin and melanin
   d. sebaceous gland and excretory tubes
   e. none of the above

5. The _____ is the surface layer of the skin.

    a. melanin
    b. epidermis
    c. dermis
    d. sebaceous gland
    e. none of the above

6. The _____ primary function is to provide nourishment to the epidermis.

    a. melanin's
    b. epidermis's
    c. dermis's
    d. excretory gland's
    e. none of the above

7. _____ is a pigment that gives skin its color and is produced in the epidermis.

    a. Melanin
    b. Epidermis
    c. Dermis
    d. Sebaceous gland
    e. None of the above

8. The _____ connects the skin to the surface muscles.

    a. sebaceous layer
    b. sudoriferous
    c. subcutaneous tissue
    d. skin appendages
    e. none of the above

9. The elastic fibers connect _____ tissue with the dermis.

   a. gland tissue
   b. sudoriferous
   c. sebaceous glands
   d. sebum
   e. all of the above

10. _____ and nerve endings are routed throughout the subcutaneous layer.

   a. Blood vessels
   b. Capillaries
   c. Nerves
   d. All of the above
   e. None of the above

11. The _____ secrete water, mineral salt, and other substances in order to help cool down the body and regulate temperature.

   a. subcutaneous layer
   b. sebaceous glands
   c. sudoriferous glands
   d. all of the above
   e. none of the above

12. The _____ are glands that secrete an oily substance.

   a. sudoriferous glands
   b. sebaceous glands
   c. subcutaneous glands
   d. all of the above
   e. none of the above

13. Glands have _____ that extend to the skin surface and open at the pores.

   a. sebum
   b. keratin
   c. excretory tubes
   d. capillaries
   e. none of the above

14. Hair can be found over most of the body although the amount of hair on each individual is _____.

   a. different
   b. the same
   c. similar
   d. equivalent
   e. none of the above

15. Hair is composed of a substance called _____.

   a. melanin
   b. sebum
   c. keratin
   d. a hair follicle
   e. none of the above

16. The sweat glands are located in the _____.

   a. melamine
   b. epidermis
   c. dermis
   d. follicles
   e. none of the above

17. A thin band of involuntary muscle is attached to most hair on the _____.

    a. sweat gland
    b. sebaceous gland
    c. excretory gland
    d. subcutaneous glands
    e. none of the above

18. The _____ system provides a protective covering for the body systems.

    a. melanin
    b. dermis
    c. integumentary
    d. subcutaneous
    e. none of the above

19. The integumentary system is composed of _____.

    a. nails
    b. sweat glands
    c. hair
    d. all of the above
    e. none of the above

20. The integumentary system protects body organs from _____.

    a. harmful substances
    b. bacteria
    c. ultraviolet rays
    d. all of the above
    e. none of the above

The Urinary System

Unit Test 8

1. The urinary or excretory system has _____ main organs.

    a. 2
    b. 4
    c. 5
    d. 10
    e. none of the above

2. The urinary system excretes body waste and excessive _____ from the body.

    a. water
    b. blood
    c. plasma
    d. all of the above
    e. none of the above

3. The human body has _____ kidneys.

    a. 1
    b. 3
    c. 4
    d. 2
    e. none of the above

4. Kidneys act as _____.

    a. cones
    b. filters
    c. hormones
    d. carrier tubes
    e. none of the above

5. _____ is the liquid waste produced and excreted from the kidney.

   a. Potassium
   b. Sodium
   c. Urine
   d. Uric acid
   e. None of the above

6. Ammonia, urea, uric acid, excessive water, potassium, sodium, and other substances are included in _____.

   a. urine
   b. blood
   c. blood cells
   d. red blood cells
   e. none of the above

7. The _____ is a tube that carries urine from the kidneys into the urinary bladder.

   a. urethra
   b. urine
   c. prostate gland
   d. ureter
   e. none of the above

8. The body has _____ ureters.

   a. 2
   b. 3
   c. 4
   d. 6
   e. none of the above

9. One _____ extends from each kidney.

    a. ureter

    b. urinary bladder

    c. urethra

    d. prostate gland

    e. none of the above

10. The ureters extend from the kidney to and through the _____.

    a. peristalsis

    b. prostate

    c. urinary bladder

    d. ureter

    e. none of the above

11. The _____ is a temporary reservoir used to hold urine.

    a. urinary bladder

    b. peristalsis

    c. ureter

    d. urethra

    e. none of the above

12. When the bladder is full of urine, it expels the urine into the _____.

    a. renal arteries

    b. urethra

    c. kidney

    d. peristalsis

    e. none of the above

13. The urethra is a _____ that extends from the bladder to the outside.

    a. gland
    b. cavity
    c. tube
    d. peristalsis
    e. none of the above

14. The bladder empties _____ into the urethra.

    a. nutrients
    b. filters
    c. hormones
    d. urine
    e. none of the above

15. The urethra expels the _____ outside the body.

    a. blood
    b. plasma
    c. nutrients
    d. all of the above
    e. none of the above

16. The urethra is _____ in both men and women.

    a. the same
    b. not included
    c. the same size
    d. all of the above
    e. none of the above

17. The urethra is part of _____ reproduction system.

    a. the female

    b. the male

    c. both male and female

    d. neither male nor female

    e. none of the above

18. The urethra is joined by two ducts that carry male _____.

    a. nutrients

    b. blood

    c. prostate glands

    d. sex cells

    e. none of the above

19. Kidney hormones help regulate _____.

    a. growth

    b. urine

    c. blood pressure

    d. reproduction

    e. none of the above

20. A low red blood cell count is called _____.

    a. anemia

    b. renal failure

    c. low blood pressure

    d. high blood pressure

    e. none of the above

The Endocrine System

Unit Test 9

1. The endocrine system consists of organs that produce _____.

    a. water
    b. hormones
    c. glands
    d. protein
    e. none of the above

2. _____ are chemical messengers that help regulate body functions.

    a. Glands
    b. Calcitonin
    c. Thyroxine
    d. Progesterone
    e. None of the above

3. Hormones are secreted by the _____ glands.

    a. phosphorous
    b. glycogen
    c. endocrine
    d. progesterone
    e. none of the above

4. The endocrine system and _____ systems are the two main systems that control and coordinate other systems of the body.

    a. respiratory
    b. nervous
    c. circulatory
    d. brain
    e. none of the above

5. There are _____ kinds of hormones.

   a. 6
   b. 2
   c. 5
   d. 10
   e. none of the above

6. _____ hormones make up most of the body's hormones.

   a. Phosphorous
   b. Steroids
   c. Calcium
   d. Protein
   e. none of the above

7. The endocrine system can be divided into _____ main gland groups.

   a. 6
   b. 5
   c. 1
   d. 2
   e. none of the above

8. The _____ glands are the largest of the endocrine glands.

   a. thyroid
   b. pituitary
   c. adrenal cortex
   d. parathyroid
   e. none of the above

9. _____, along with other growth hormones, promotes normal growth.

    a. Glucocorticoid
    b. Epinephrine
    c. Progesterone
    d. Thyroxine
    e. none of the above

10. The _____ glands secrete the parathyroid hormone.

    a. adrenal
    b. adrenal cortex
    c. parathyroid
    d. pituitary
    e. none of the above

11. The _____ acts to promote the release of calcium from the bone tissue into the bloodstream.

    a. adrenal
    b. adrenal cortex
    c. pituitary
    d. parathyroid gland
    e. none of the above

12. The _____ glands are divided into two parts.

    a. thyroid
    b. adrenal
    c. pituitary
    d. parathyroid
    e. none of the above

13. _____ acts as a neurotransmitter.

   a. Epinephrine
   b. Glucocorticoid
   c. Thyroxine
   d. Testosterone
   e. none of the above

14. _____ is a hormone produced by the adrenal medulla glands that regulate blood pressure.

   a. Thyroxine
   b. Epinephrine
   c. Testosterone
   d. Glucocorticoid
   e. None of the above

15. The _____ glands secrete two main hormones.

   a. pituitary
   b. parathyroid
   c. thyroid
   d. adrenal cortex
   e. none of the above

16. _____ are hormones that suppress inflammatory responses.

   a. Epinephrines
   b. Glucocorticoids
   c. Thyroxines
   d. Testosterones
   e. None of the above

17. _____ regulate the body's electrolyte balance.

    a. Glucocorticoids

    b. Pancreas

    c. Adrenal cortex

    d. Neurotransmitters

    e. None of the above

18. The _____ secretes the hormones glucagon and insulin.

    a. brain

    b. thyroid glands

    c. adrenal cortex

    d. pancreas

    e. none of the above

19. Testosterone is the main _____ sex hormone.

    a. male and female

    b. female

    c. male

    d. super

    e. none of the above

20. The _____ glands are controlled by the nervous system.

    a. thyroid

    b. pituitary

    c. adrenal

    d. parathyroid

    e. none of the above

Individualized Shadowing Evaluation Worksheet

Date	Assignment					
Student	Location					
Evaluator	Outstanding	Excellent	Above average	Passing	Needs work	Phone number
Coverage area	1	2	3	4	5	Notes
Dress						
Communication skills						
Punctuality						
Following instructions						
Professionalism						
Initiative						
Cooperation						
Interpersonal skills						
Willingness to learn						
Ability to learn						

Total score   Grade

50-45 = A

44-40 = B

39-30 = C

29-20 = D

19-10 = No Pass

Introductory Health Science

Phase 2
Basic Health Concerns

1. Goals and Purpose
    The student will

    a. develop a general concept of the broad scope of the discipline of health science;
    b. become familiar with importance of diet and nutrition;
    c. learn the names and *dangers* of commonly known communicable diseases;
    d. develop a basic understanding of sanitation, disinfection, and sterilization and learn of available immunizations and methods for preventing diseases and illnesses;
    e. become familiar with common health concerns for men;
    f. become familiar with common health concerns for women;
    g. become *knowledgeable* of the signs, symptoms, and adverse effects of alcohol, tobacco, and drug addiction;
    h. receive training in emergency first aid treatment including CPR;
    i. learn the basic supplies and equipment needed in every home to make a home health center.

2. Performance Objective
    This phase consists of ten units. For each unit, the student will

    a. read the instructor-developed packet for the concept/s being taught,
    b. actively participate in lectures,

    c. complete the packet worksheet/s with accuracy,

    d. pass the instructor-made test with a minimum,

    e. pass the terminology quiz with a minimum score of 80% or better.

3. Instructional Strategy

    The instructional strategies will include the use of various acknowledged teaching procedures including general lectures, class discussions, concept quizzes, objectives testing, demonstrations, individualized instructions, group instructions, and when possible, guest speakers will be utilized. Audio and video materials will also be used when applicable and available. Students will be encouraged to read outside materials covering the concepts being taught. Each section will include reading materials, vocabulary builders, a unit quiz, a vocabulary quiz, and instructor-led lectures/discussions.

4. Times of Instruction and Major Units of Instruction Hours

    A. Course Description and Preparation

        Unit 1: Introduction to Health Science

        Unit 2: Immunization and Prevention

        Unit 3: Basic Nutrition

        Unit 4: Communicable Diseases

        Unit 5: Sanitation, Disinfection, and Sterilization

        Unit 6: Alcohol, Tobacco, and Drug Addiction

        Unit 7: Women's Health

        Unit 8: Men's Health

        Unit 9: First Aid and Emergencies

        Unit 10: Developing a Self-Care Home Health Center

B. Final Test

5. Method of Evaluation

   A. Evaluation will consist of the following:

      a. 1 unit test (20 questions each)
      b. 1 unit terminology test (20 questions each)
      c. 1 final evaluation test (100 questions)

   B. Students who complete this phase will achieve the following:

      a. A minimum score of 75% on each unit terminology test and an average score of 80% on the eight test
      b. A minimum score of 75% on each unit terminology test and an average of 80% on the eight test
      c. A minimum score of 80% on the final 100-question test

Sabrina Hutton Edmond

Name _____

Date _____

Crossword Puzzle
Excretion

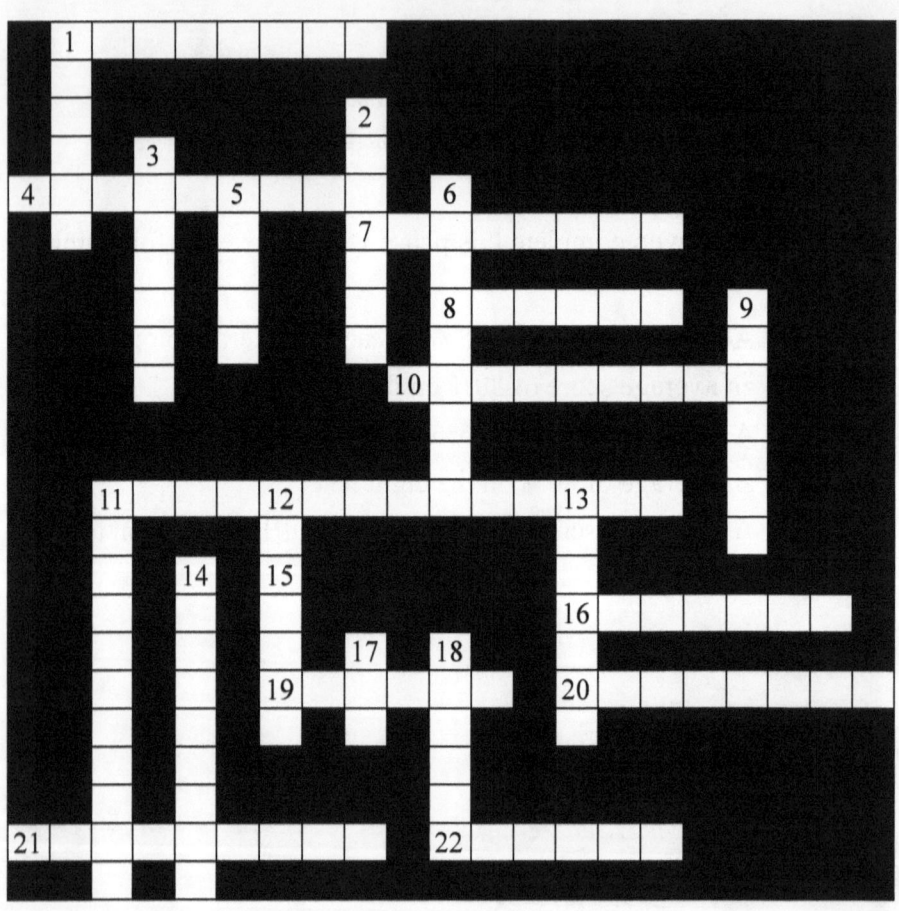

Across

1. Inflammation of the urinary bladder
4. Inflammation of the liver
7. Accessory organ of the digestive tract that produces insulin and pancreatic enzymes
8. Enzyme produced in the stomach that helps breakdown fats
10. Bloody urine
11. The filtering unit of the kidney; the beginning of the nephron
15. Finger-like projections in the intestines; contain capillaries
16. Windpipe; from the larynx to the stomach
19. Voice box; located between the pharynx and the trachea
20. Inflammation of the nasal cavity lining
21. Respiratory disease caused by pathogens; infection producing microorganisms
22. Lung disease, bronchial spasm or excessive fluid of the mucosal.

Down

1. The outer layer of the kidney; contains most of the nephrons
2. Difficult or painful breathing
3. Kidney stones; made up of uric acid and calcium salts
5. Last section of the small intestine that empties through the ileocecal valve
6. Highly communicable disease of the upper respiratory tract
9. The throat; containing three sections
11. The smaller portion of the bronchial tubes that enter into the alveoli
12. Tiny air sac in the lungs where the gas exchange occurs
13. The tube that transports urine from the bladder out of the body
14. Chronic irreversible disease that affects the gas exchange in the alveoli causing trapped air
17. Abbreviation for upper respiratory infection
18. Absence of oxygen

Name _____

Date _____

Crossword Puzzle

Support, Movement, and Protection

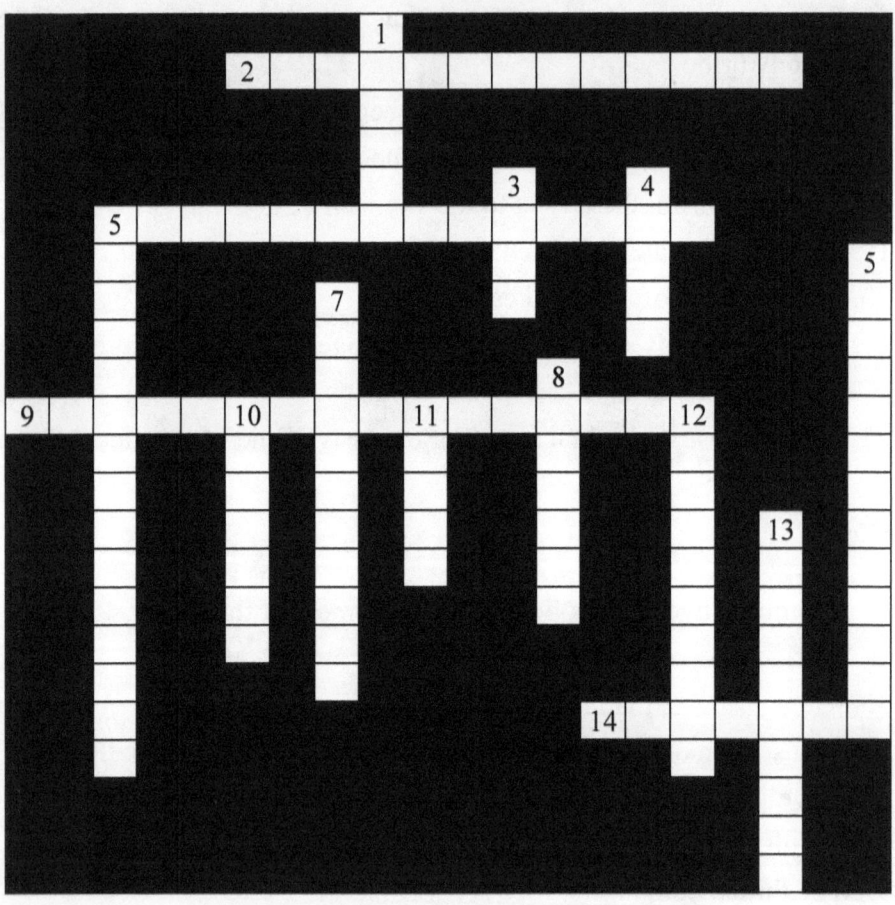

Across

2. Able to selectively permit substances to enter and exit the cell
5. Fibrous tissue located at the distal part of the calf muscle
9. A substance that supports and connects parts to each other
14. The science that deals with the body structure

Down

1. Make larger
3. The basic unit of life
4. A place where two or more bones meet
5. A term for the digestive tract
6. The skin and its appendages
7. Rhythmic motion in the digestive tract
8. Bone tissue
9. Make smaller
10. Pertaining to the heart
11. Excessive fluid in the tissues
12. Tissue that lines the cavities of the body
13. The science that deals with body function

Body Systems 3

			¹M	U	S	²C	L	E	T	I	S	S	U	E
						O								
³E		⁴O	R	G	A	N	S	Y	S	T	E	M	S	
P						N								
I		⁵N	E	R	V	E	T	I	S	S	U	E		
T						C								
⁶H	O	M	E	⁷O	S	T	A	S	I	S				
E				R		S				⁸N				
L				G		⁹T	I	S	S	U	E	S		
I				A		I				R				
A				N		S				V				
L				S		S				O				
						U				U				
¹⁰H	O	R	M	O	N	E	S			S				

Across

1. contracts or shorten
4. group of organs
5. con-chem messenger
6. ext. int. balance
9. group of cells
10. chemical messengers

Down

2. supports and connect
3. outside protectant
7. group of tissue
8. sensation

Medical prefixes & suffix

										¹P
	²T	O	M	A		³S	U	⁴B		E
	R						E	N	⁵P	O	D
	A						N	A			
	⁷I	N	T	R	A		⁸D	E	N	T	
⁹H		S		¹⁰C	I	S	E		H		
Y		¹¹T	T			R					
¹²O	P	H	T	H	A	L	M	¹³M	A	L	
E		E	Y								
R		R									
	¹⁴H	E	M	A							
	Y										
	¹⁵P	O	S	T							
¹⁶B	I	O									

Across

16. Life

teeth

bad
blood
after

Down

1. child
2. across
4. good
5. disease
6. hands
8. skin
9. eyes
11. hear
14. under

Sabrina's Anatomy Puzzle

		¹C	I	²R	C	U	L	A	T	O	R	Y		³A
				E										N
	⁴E	S	O	P	H	A	G	U	S		⁵N			A
				R					⁶H	E	A	R		T
				O							R			O
				⁷D	I	G	E	S	T	I	V	E		M
				U							O			Y
	⁸M	U	S	C	U	L	A	R			U		⁹K	
				T						¹⁰S	K	I	N
¹¹R	E	S	P	I	T	O	R	Y		¹²O			D
				V					¹³B	R	A	I	N
¹⁴S	K	E	L	E	T	A	L			G			E
										A			Y
										N			

Across

1. What carries blood
4. Digestive System
6. What is a Powerful pump
7. What breaks down food
8. blow body movement
9. Epidermis, Dermis
10. What expels Carbon Dioxide
11. What is considered Human Computer
13. The bodies framework

Down

2. Cont. Ovary Thymus
3. Study of the body
5. Contains the Born
9. Removes body waste
12. Form body systems

Body Systems 2

	¹R	E	S	P	²I	R	A	T	O	R	Y		
					N								
³E	X	⁴C	R	E	T	A	R	Y			⁵M		
N		I			E			⁶T			U		
D		R			G		⁷C	I			S		
O		C			U		E	S		⁸D	C		
C		U			M		L	S		I	U		
R		L			E		L	U		G	L		
I		A			N	⁹S	K	E	L	E	T	A	L
N		T			T			S		S	R		
E		O			A					T			
	¹⁰R	E	P	R	O	D	U	C	T	I	O	N	
	Y			Y						V			
				¹¹I	M	M	U	N	E				

Across	Down
From oxygen to O2	2. regulate temperature
what removes waste	3. regulates
what protects, supports	4. transport nutrients
What are sex functions	5. allows movement
What system fights diseases	6. group of cell
	7. building_____.
	8. absorbs nutrients

Career Planning

Name _____

Date _____

Career Planning—Puzzle 1

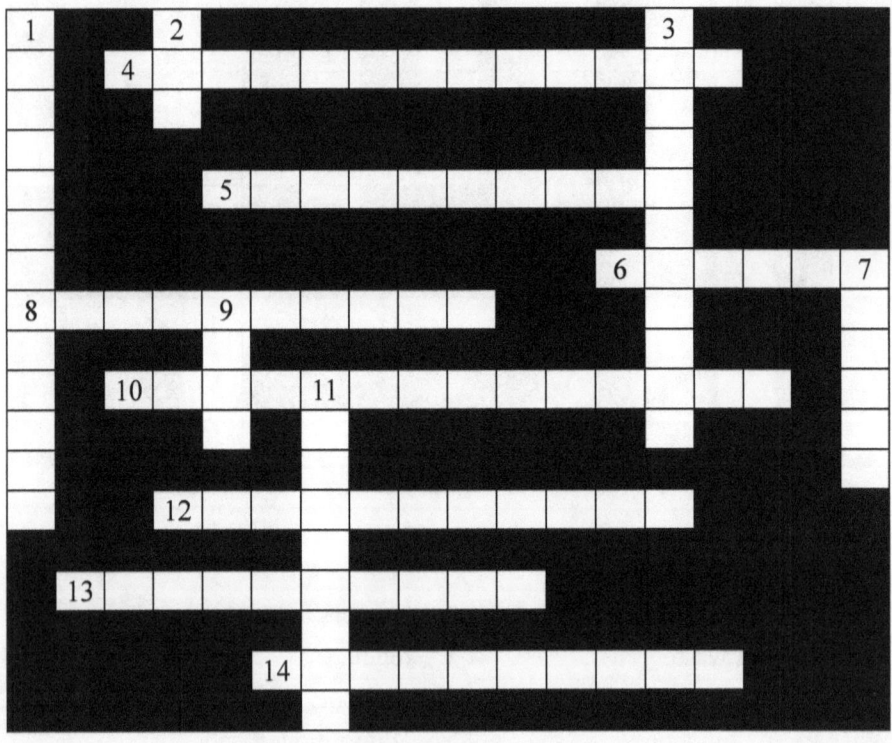

Across

4. Verbal or nonverbal exchange of messages, thoughts, ideas, and feelings
5. The drive to first begin an action
6. A profession for which one trains and that is undertaken as one's lifelong work
8. Related to past experience, knowledge, or education
10. Characteristics which make a person fit for a job
12. A piece of writing that accompanies a resume to explain or introduce its contents (2 words)
13. The way one looks, including clothes, growing habits, local expressions
14. The number of times a person is present or available to perform certain obligation at work

Down

1. The degree of reliance or trust that can be placed in a person
2. A specific role that is performed regularly for compensation
3. Working together in a harmonious fashion to accomplish a goal
7. A brief written account of personal and professional qualifications and experience
9. Something desired and to which an effort is made
11. Honesty

Introduction to Medical Terminology

Name _____

Date _____

Introduction to Medical Terminology—Puzzle 1

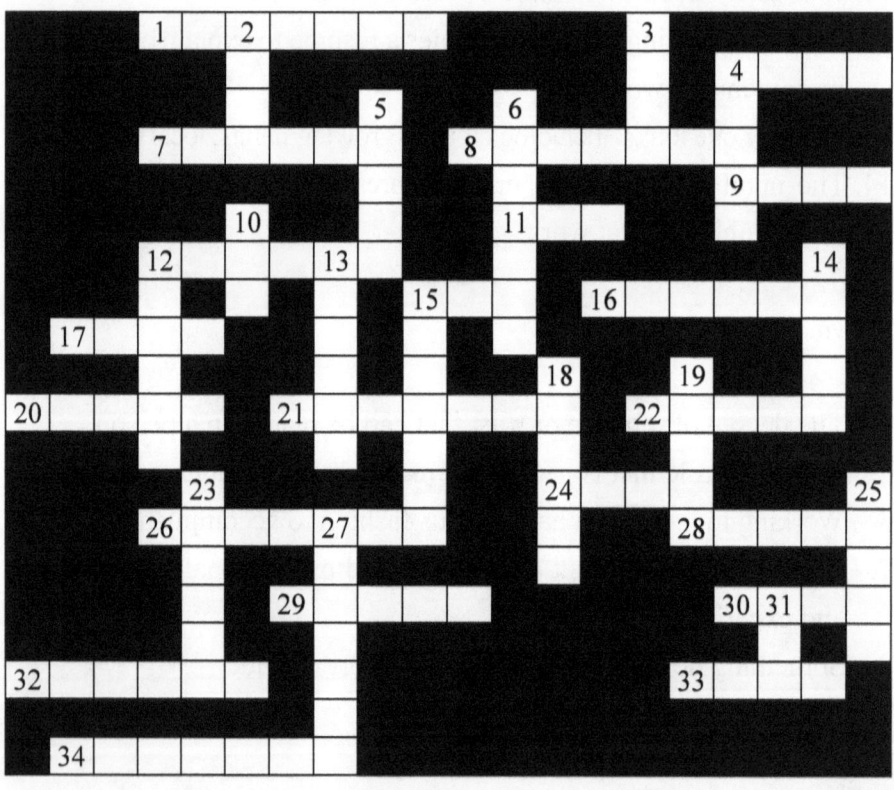

Across

1. Dilation, expansion, or stretching
4. Half or partial
7. Twisted
8. Head
9. Many
11. Upon, over, or upper
12. False
15. Three
16. Excessive flow
17. Record
20. Near
21. Arm
22. White
24. Against
26. Viscera, internal organs
28. Vessel, either blood or lymph
29. Blue
30. Pushing or driving away
32. Surgical removal, excision
33. The ilium, part of hip bone
34. Pertaining to the meninges.

Down

2. Order, arrangement or coordination
3. Enlarged
4. Visual examination
5. Rib
6. Movement
10. Blood
12. Surgical repair
13. Right side
14. Lips
15. Windpipe
18. The body
19. Lack of or deficiency
23. Surrounding or around
25. Alike or the same
27. Red
31. One

Infection Control

Name _____

Date _____

Infection Control—Puzzle 1

Across

???

Down

???

Understanding the Patient as a Person

Name _____

Date _____

Understanding the Patient as a Person—Puzzle 1

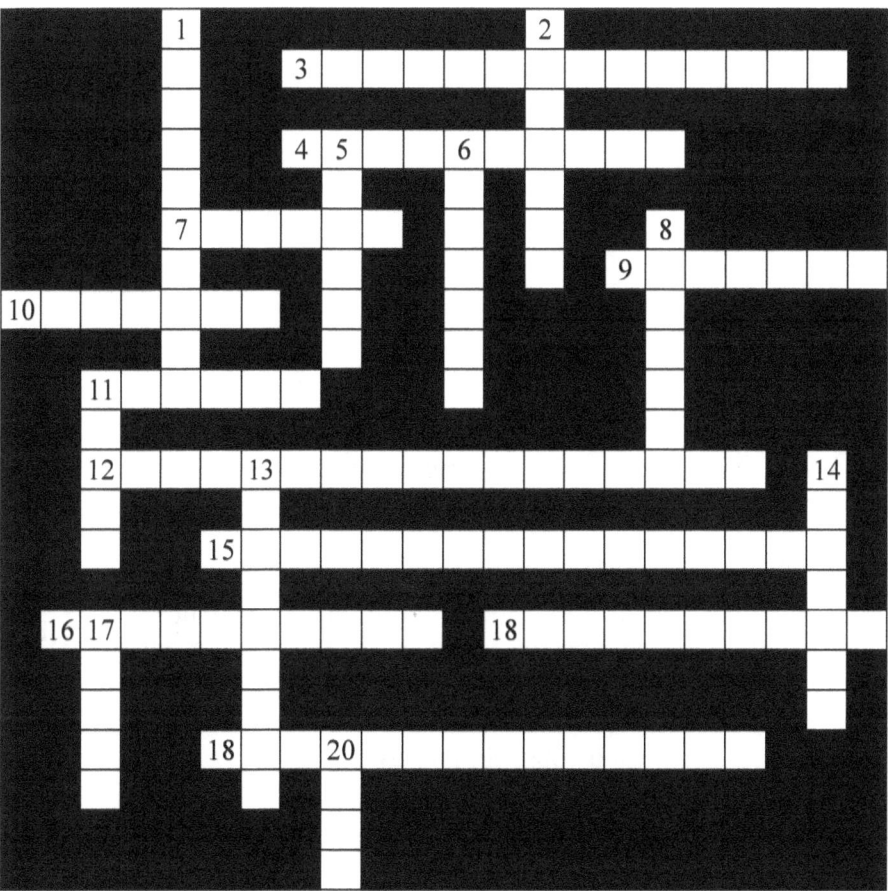

Across

1. Excessive use of chemicals, drugs, or alcohol??? Words
4. Final stage of the dying process
7. When events or circumstances challenge ??? one's coping mechanisms
9. The skills and arts of a given people_____.
10. The voluntary ending of one's life
11. The first stage of the dying process
12. Causes irreversible memory loss and physical detectors _____ commonly seen in late adulthood 2 words
13. The methods by which an individual

Down

1. The fourth stage of the dying process
2. Describes babies from birth to 1 year of age
5. A _____ practice or a particular people _____ group
6. When males and females become capable of reproduction
8. A mental illness characterized by overeating binges followed by voluntary vomiting fasting or _____ diarrhea
11. The _____ of life as indicated by the permanent _____ of all vital functions
13. _____ to one's feelings.
14. _____ care and counseling to dying.

Basic First Aid

Name _____

Date _____

Basic First Aid—Puzzle 1

238 Sabrina Hutton Edmond

Across

3. See 6 Down
4. An injury to soft tissue in which a flap of tissue is torn loose or pulled off
10. An injury to the soft tissues of a joint, characterized by pain, deformity, and the inability to move
12. Describes a patient who is perspiring profusely
14. A maneuver for open_____ a blocked airway 4 words
17. Drawing in by suck_____

Down

1. Facing sudden, brief loss of consciousness
2. The black and blue color caused by seepage of blood into tissue as in a confusion
5. A neurological dysfunction that may result in involuntary uncontrolled muscle contractions
6. A heart attack; a condition caused by the blockage of one or more coronary arteries with ???
7. The absence of a heartbeat (2 words)
8. An emetic used to induce vomiting (3 words)
9. The immediate care provided to a person involved in a medical emergency (2 words)
11. Tissue death caused by a lack of oxygen
13. A maneuver used to open the airway in a neck-injured patient (2 words)
15. Poisonous
16. Method used to turn a patient with suspected spinal injury (2 words)

Excretion

Name _____

Date _____

Excretion—Puzzle 1

Across

3. A lack of oxygen
7. The throat
8. Difficult or painful breathing, shortness of breath
10. The tube that transports urine from the bladder
13. A corpuscle at the end of a nephron that contains the glomerulus (2 words)
18. Upper respiratory infection
19. What is a tube of cartilage extending from the thoraic in the brochi tubes
23. Inflammation of the lining of the nasal cavity
24. The presence of blood urinary

Down

1. Inflammation of the lungs
2. The organ that produces enzymes and aids in digestion
4. The voice box
5. An enzyme that breaks down fats
6. A highly communicable disease of the upper respiratory tract
9. Smaller portion of the
11. Inflammation of the liver
12. The last section of the small intestine
14. Inflammation of the urinary bladder
15. A chronic lung disease that destroys the alveoli
16. Finger-like projections found on membrane surfaces
17. Stones usually made up of minerals salts
20. Microscopic air sacs in the lungs
21. The outer layer of an organ such as the kidney
22. Causes breathing difficulty, wheezing, and coughing

The Safe Workplace

Name _____

Date _____

The Safe Workplace—Puzzle 1

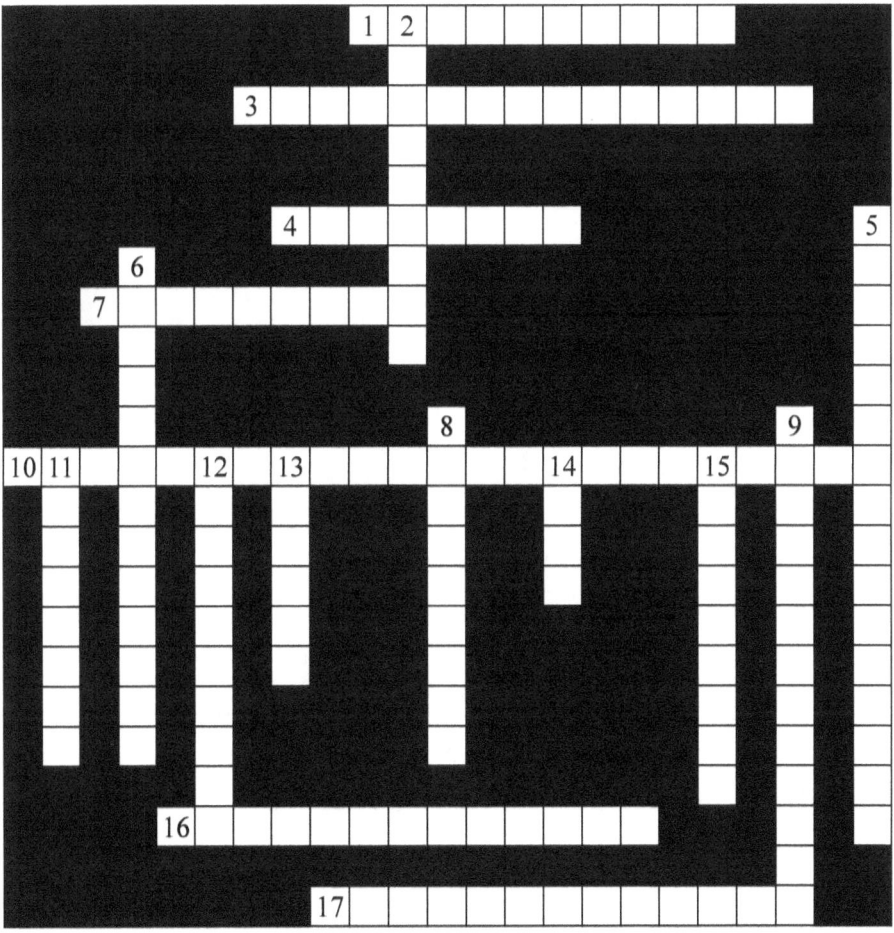

Across

1. A jagged tear in the flesh
3. The basic lifesaving procedure that is done in the event of a cardiac arrest; with 9 Down
4. A substance capable of causing injury either through direct contact on the skin or by the inhalation of gaseous fumes
7. A soft tissue injury caused by seepage of blood into tissue; a bruise
10. An official document that identifies all the chemicals used in a specific department (4 words)
16. An extreme stimulation of the nerves by the passage of current through the body (2 words)
17. The extent to which a joint can _____.

Down

2. The positioning of parts in a straight line
5. A canister filled with chemicals to combat different types of fires (2 words)
6. The efficient and safe use of the body during activity (2 words)
8. Pertaining to the upper portion of the spine
9. Revive or bring back to life; See 3 Across
11. An unforeseen, unfortunate occurrence; See 12 Down
12. An injury sustained while working; with 11 Down
13. The lower back between the thorax and the pelvis
14. A cartilaginous cushion between the vertebrae
15. Devices on a bed of gurney used to prevent a patient fall

Disasters: Preparedness, Hazards, and Prevention

Name _____
Date _____

Disasters: Preparedness, Hazards, and Prevention—Puzzle 1

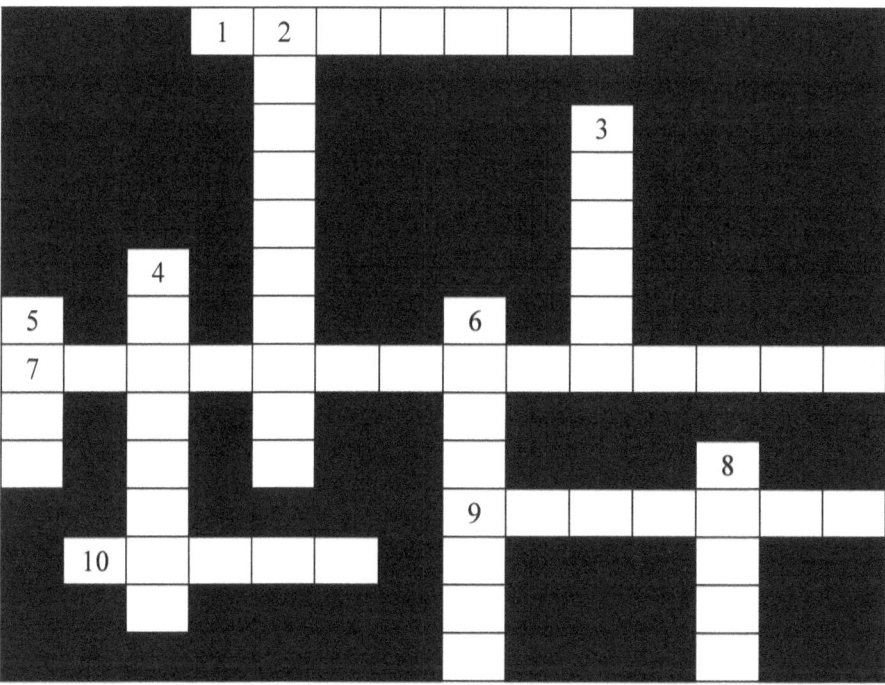

244   Sabrina Hutton Edmond

Across

1. Potentially dangerous or deadly conditions existing in a workplace
7. Information provided by a patient about their _____ experience (2 words)
9. Not able to produce children
10. Poisonous

Down

2. An evaluation of a patient's condition
3. To _____ prioritize care for a group of patients
4. A form of magnesium and calcium silicate formerly used in construction and for fireproofing
5. Abbreviation for Occupational Safety and Health Administration
6. An unexpected event that causes great damage and depletes _____ exhausts currently available resources
8. Abbreviation of National Institute for _____ and Health

Bibliography

Bailey, Donna. *Health Facts Series*. 8 vols. Austin Steck-Vaughn, 1991.

Catherall, Ed. *Exploring the Human Body*. Austin Steck-Vaughn, 1992.

Gerard, J. Tortora. *Principles of Human Anatomy*. 6th ed. New York: Harper Collins, 1992.

Hollinshead, W. H., and C. Rosse. *Textbook of Anatomy*. 4th ed. Philadelphia: J. B. Lippincott, 1985.

Memmler, Ruth L., Barbara Janson-Cohen, and Dena Lin Wood. *The Human Body in Health and Disease*. 7th ed. Philadelphia: J. B. Lippincott Company, 1992.

Netler, F. H. *Musculoskeletal System: Anatomy, Physiology, and Metabolic Disorders*. Summit, NJ: CIBA, 1987.

Shipman, P., A. Walker, and D. Bichell. *The Human Skeleton*. Cambridge: Harvard University Press, 1985.

Index